Autophagy:

Live healthy. Discover your self-cleansing body's natural intelligence! Activate the anti-aging process through the ketosis state, extended water, intermittent fasting, and ketogenic diet!

by

Serena Baker

Table of Contents

Introduction

The human body is a vast universe of intelligence. We often forget how sophisticated our internal machinery is, and our daily lives were spent focusing on the external results. So much of our life-long health is determined by what goes on inside on a microscopic level. What you cannot see going on inside of you is immense. Every meal you eat, every beverage you drink, and every moment of rest or exertion have a lasting impact on your internal machinery.

All of us are looking for the right diet, exercise routine, and prescription drug to make us look and feel good for all of our lives. We sport the latest fad diet, intending to get healthier, energized, or lose weight, and we concentrate only on our fitness regimens as our way of supporting a long, healthy life, free of disease and chronic illness. All of these things contribute to something much deeper. With the right intake of food, exercise, and an occasional break from both, your body begins to experience autophagy.

Over time, our cells produce by-products and waste from the hard work that they are constantly doing. This microscopic bio-waste is collected in the cell, like an overflowing trash can. This happens when we eat too many sugars and carbohydrates, changing our insulin absorption and affecting our whole system's ability to function properly. When the cells are running slow because the waste is building up on account of a poor diet, lack of exercise, and our over-consumption of food daily, slowly over time, we begin to see the results: cancer, diabetes, inflammatory disease, cardiovascular disease, and rapid aging.

Our bodies are intelligent and know how to clean house and heal, especially if we create the right conditions for this process to occur. Autophagy is a self-healing mechanism at the cellular level that when achieved can change the health of your whole life. This book is an instruction manual, giving you guidance about what it is and how it works, why and when to activate it, and what results you can expect from autophagy performance.

Your health is in your hands all the way down to your cells. Begin your healing journey now!

Chapter 1: Understanding Autophagy

You may already have a basic understanding on the way the body works—blood, muscles, and bones—operated by a computer called the brain that sends information throughout the body to allow it to operate. We have systems for everything: digestion, breathing, going to the bathroom, and reproducing. Every part of us is a system, and those systems are built with cells. The basic building block of every person starts with a tiny, little machine with its own set of rules and orders.

In order to understand autophagy, you must consider the cell and how trillions of them create your everyday being. They all function individually, as part of a whole system and finally as a whole working human body. Like all living things, there are types of organisms that we all have inside of us, like microbes, bacteria, free radicals, and viruses that cannot function unless all of our cells are running on a healthy level. Some of these things such as microbes and certain bacteria are good and wanted in the system, while other forms of bacteria, free radicals, and viruses are what we want our cells to fight off and destroy. How can our cells effectively fight anything if they are unhealthy?

Fighting against all of the illnesses, diseases, inflammations, and other concerns of our health is the work of the cell. Right now, in our society, there is a huge lack of understanding about how we all give ourselves the toxins and poisons that create cell dysfunction, that leads to illness and loss of life. The reason why we all have diseases is because we are giving it to ourselves, through our foods, drinks, lack of exercise, processed foods, chemicals, and pollution.

If you want a healthy, long life, you have to understand the internal partnership of your cells and your overall well-being. It's not a matter of what drug you can take to fix the problem quickly, or what surgery can be performed to extract disease. Health and wellness begin inside, on a deep, cellular level. We cannot expect to feel well if we do not heal from this microscopic point of view. The chronic plague of cancer, diabetes, neurodegenerative illnesses, and all the inflammatory disorders and dysfunctions come from one, significant point: the health of the cell.

There are reasons for poor health and poor physical performance that stem from the ability or lack of ability for your cells to clean themselves or eat-away at the biowaste that comes naturally to a hard-working organism. This ability is autophagy.

Autophagy is very simply put as cell function. It is a normal occurrence that allows for the proper recycling of material. There are specific functions in every cell, based on what part of the body or system they operate in. Some are muscle cells, others make up your brain, while several are responsible for the building up and breaking down of bone.

We don't behave in our lives, thinking about how and what we do to affect these tiny, little parts of us. We tend to view life from the macroscopic point of view; it is in our nature to do so. There is so much occurring every moment that we cannot see or feel. Knowing and understanding how our bodies function at a cellular level is the key to healing ourselves.

Beginning your course in understanding autophagy starts with the basics. To know autophagy, you have to know the cell and how it functions.

Ch 1.1: The What and How of Autophagy

Autophagy, when broken down, translates from Greek to mean "self-eating." This is a normal, biological process in the human body that occurs on the cellular level, deep within the cytoplasm. Breaking down the cell and its components can shed more light on why autophagy occurs in the first place.

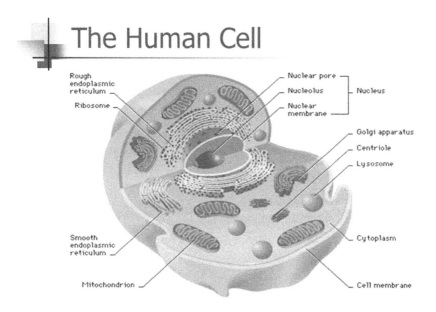

The basic cell of any human is made of proteins, lipids, cholesterol, and water, and these components make up the mechanisms that encourage healthy cell performance.

A cell is a sophisticated machine comprised of many organelles, plasma, amino acids, glucose, genetic information, and chemical compounds that help the cell to perform its functions. Here is a breakdown of what you will find within every cell in the body, no matter what body system it is working in:

Nucleus

- The nucleus has a double membrane and is a spherical shape containing your DNA strands. This part of the cells dictates protein synthesis, playing a major role in our cell performance, most specifically active transport of genetic information, metabolism, growth, and heredity.

Nucleoli

- A dense region, and part of the nucleus, the nucleoli play a major part in the creation of ribosomes.

Ribosome

- Tiny particles in the cell made of rRNA sub-particles. The job of the ribosome is to synthesize proteins. It is often referred to as the protein factory of the cell.

Cilia

- These are short, hair-like extensions on the outer surface of the cell that can move substances or particles over the outer surface.

Plasma Membrane

- This is the phospholipid layer of the skin of the cell. It is studded with proteins and serves as the cell's gatekeeper, the castle wall. When there are carbohydrates and proteins on the outer side of the cell, they will perform certain functions connected to the plasma membrane such as allowing for individual cell identification as a receptor for certain hormones, like the gatekeepers at the gate.

Mitochondria

- This organelle is a network of membranous folds covered in enzymes and is where your ATP, or adenosine triphosphate, is synthesized. They are referred to as the cell powerhouses, creating energy on the microscopic level for the whole body.

Lysosomes

- A round, bubble-like organelle, covered in a membrane, the lysosome is the digestive system or recycling center of the cell.

Centrioles

- A pair of hollow cylinders made up of tiny tubules, the function of the centriole is cell reproduction.

Golgi Apparatus

- A stack of flat, membranous sacs, the Golgi apparatus chemically processes and packages substances from the endoplasmic reticulum.

Endoplasmic Reticulum (ER)

- There is rough ER and smooth ER. Rough ER is covered in ribosomes, while smooth ER has no attached organelles. The ER is a network of sacs and canals and has a membranous quality.

Every human cell performs certain functions. Some functions of the cell are to maintain its own survival, and other functions are to maintain the body's survival. Most of the time, the number and type of organelles allow the cells to differ dramatically regarding how they specifically function. For example, cells that contain a large number of mitochondria, such as cardiovascular muscle cells, are capable of sustained work. The excess of mitochondria can synthesize more ATP to have more energy in the cell; they can support the necessary energy required for ongoing rhythmic contractions. Movement of the flagellum of sperm, the only cell in the body to have a flagellum (tail), is another example of a specialized organelle and its specific function. The sperm, a cell in the male reproductive system, is propelled by the flagellum through the reproductive tract of the female, increasing the chances of fertilization. Every cell has a distinct purpose and health.

All cells require some movement bringing things in and pushing things out. The movement of substances through cells is a major aspect of our ability to live healthfully. If our cells reject nutrient because they are unable to absorb any, then you and your cells will suffer.

The plasma membrane in a healthy cell separates the contents of the cell from the tissue fluid that surrounds it. At the same time, the membrane has to permit certain substances and chemical compounds to enter the cell and allow others to depart. Heavy traffic moves continuously in both directions through all cell membranes. Things like water molecules, food molecules, gases, wastes, and many others flow in and out of cells in an endless procession. There are two general ways this process occurs: *passive* and *active* transport processes.

Active transport requires the expenditure of energy by the cell; passive transport does not. The energy required for the active transport process is obtained through ATP or adenosine triphosphate. ATP is created in the mitochondria of the cell, using energy from nutrients, and is capable of releasing that energy to do work within the cell. For active transport to occur, the breakdown of ATP and use of that released energy are required.

The details of active and passive transport are much easier to understand if you remember two key facts:

1. Passive transport—no cellular energy is required to move substances from a high to a low concentration.

2. Active transport—cellular energy is required to move substances from a low to a high concentration.

Within each kind of transport, you can break it down further to understand the function of the cell and how it operates to stay healthy, and perform the various functions that work to keep the body alive. For example, within passive transport processes, there is diffusion, which includes osmosis and dialysis and filtration; within active transport processes, there is the ion pump, phagocytosis, and pinocytosis.

Active transport processes are what autophagy explains. Phagocytosis is most closely linked to the concept of autophagy. Autophagy is similar in that is the eating of materials within the cell. And like the transport processes, autophagy has its own variations that you will read about in the next chapter.

Bringing these concepts into a frame, consider the process of autophagy from the perspective of the lysosome.

The *lysosome* is the part of the cell to pay particular attention to when learning and understanding autophagy. It has the nickname "digestive bags" in some biological documents because of its particular job within the cell. They contain the enzymes that digest food substances. It isn't just food that they digest; they are also responsible for the digestion of microbes that invade the cell, and waste materials collected in the cell that need to be removed. Lysosomes protect the cell against destruction; they are also, in a way, the immune system of the cell.

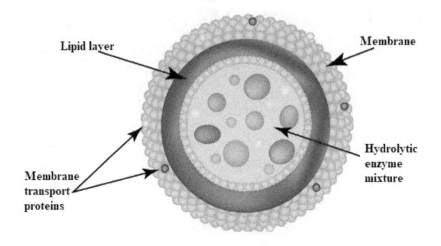

Lipid layer

Membrane

Membrane transport proteins

Hydrolytic enzyme mixture

Lysosome

The lysosome searches for pieces and parts of old, worn down, and discarded cell material, such as dead organelles, damaged proteins, oxidized particles, and other bio-waste. The cells absorb the waste matter and collect useful components to build new cell parts. It is essentially your body's recycling system that occurs on a microscopic level. This process is what allows the body to eliminate faulty, errant organisms, a cancerous growth, and cell metabolism dysfunction.

Autophagy is not to be confused with apoptosis, which is the death of the entire cell. Apoptosis is normal and occurs as a part of cell growth and development. Autophagy is the removal of dead or dysfunctional bio-matter in the cell, some of which is recycled and repaired for future use, rather than overall death of the whole machine. It is the body's system for cleaning house. Unlike our own digestive system, our cells cannot simply flush their waste down the toilet.

This process is also known to assist in your body's ability to have strong immunity and fight inflammation which can lead to a variety of health issues. Some inflammation is beneficial to your body, as when you are fighting a cold or healing from an acute wound, however, regular existence of inflammation in your body can break down your cellular function and lead to dysfunction. When you break it down, autophagy is our body's way of keeping us healthy, cancer-free, fit, energized, mentally well, and living longer. It is an adaptive response in the face of all stress.

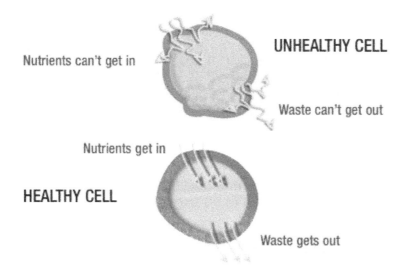

Nutrients can't get in

UNHEALTHY CELL

Waste can't get out

Nutrients get in

HEALTHY CELL

Waste gets out

When cells are stressed, such as lacking nutrients, energy, insulin, or become damaged from chronic variations of all of the above, a stress response occurs which initiates autophagy. It may seem counter-intuitive, but our cell's functioning improves when we are in a state of stress—healthy stress, of course.

What is healthy stress? Exercise, fasting, and ketosis. Without this kind of healthy stress, our cells will perform moderately and not optimally, suggesting that if you want to induce a serious, healing change in your body, you need to induce autophagy with the appropriate stress.

Autophagy is considered beneficial for many reasons, including the rejuvenation of the cells to impact life-long health and balance. When your cells age the machinery within, the cell also ages and becomes dysfunctional or nonfunctional. Autophagy is a biological maneuver to refresh and renew the cell by eliminating waste or recycling it for more efficient use and performance. By this method of cellular repair, the idea is that you can activate autophagy intentionally to promote cell rejuvenation that will reduce chances of certain age-related illnesses, diseases, and disorders. It can also repair existing conditions like diabetes, obesity, and food and health-related disorders that are the result of poor diet and lack of exercise. Several studies have shown improvement in neurodegenerative disorders, too, such as Parkinson's and Alzheimer's.

Think of it like the cell-cleansing garbage disposal crew. We have our own self-cleaning system when our cells are dirty with a build-up of old waste. It can represent in the way we feel and even the way we look. If you have dry, flaky skin and limp damaged hair, it may be due to the cell clutter that hasn't been able to clean for some reason. If you are fatigued, overweight, and aching all over, it may be because your cells cannot perform optimally under those conditions. Looking deeper into the cell will tell you more about the functions of autophagy.

Functions of Autophagy

Nutrient Starvation

Autophagy has roles in a variety of cellular functions. In yeasts, for example, the nutrient starvation activates a high level of autophagy. This permits unneeded proteins to be broken down and amino acids to be recycled for the synthesis of proteins that are necessary for survival. Autophagy is induced in higher eukaryotes in response to the nutrient depletion that occurs at birth when the trans-placental food supply is cut off, as well as that of nutrient-starved cultured cells and tissues. In nutrition-deficient conditions, Mutant yeast cells that have a reduced autophagic capability rapidly cease to be. Studies suggest that autophagy is indispensable for protein degradation in the vacuoles under fasting conditions and that around 15 APG genes are involved in autophagy in yeast. The gene ATG7 has been implicated in nutrient-mediated autophagy; starvation-induced autophagy was impaired in *atg7*-deficient mice.

Xenophagy

Xenophagy is the autophagic degradation of infectious particles. Our innate immunity is dependent upon our cellular autophagic machinery. Intracellular pathogens, like the bacterium which is responsible for tuberculosis, are chosen for degradation by the same cellular machinery and regulatory mechanisms that choose host mitochondria for mortification. This is further evidence for the endosymbiotic hypothesis, an evolutionary theory of origin. This process leads to the destruction of the invasive microorganisms; however, some bacteria can halt the maturing process of phagosomes. Activating autophagy help overcome infected cells, restoring pathogen degradation.

Infection

In the same family as the rabies virus, vesicular stomatitis virus is taken up by the autophagosome and translocated to the lysosomes, where detection of certain gene codes through a receptor occurs. After the activation of the receptor, intracellular signaling is initiated, inducing interferon and other antiviral cytokines. Viruses and bacteria subvert the autophagic pathway to promote their own replication. A protein known as Galectin-8 has recently been called an intracellular receptor for dangerous particles, capable of initiating autophagy to protect against intracellular pathogens. Galectin-8 binds to a damaged vacuole or organelle and then enlists an autophagy adaptor, leading to the formation of an autophagosome.

Repair

Autophagy deteriorates damaged cell matter such as oxidized proteins, damaged organelles, and another biowaste. Dysfunctional autophagy is considered one of the main reasons for the accumulation of damaged cells and aging.

Apoptosis

The appearance of autophagosomes can be an indicator of programmed cell death or apoptosis and depends on autophagy proteins. Autophagy is not the death of a cell; it is the renewal; however, within certain conditions, an internal cell death happens, and certain byproducts are collected and consumed. There has been confusion between apoptosis and cell and autophagy and whether they are linked. There has been a suggestion that autophagy causes cell death; however, autophagic performance in dying cells is actually an attempt to prevent the death of the cell.

Allowing your understanding of autophagy to form through all of the data and research can help you see the effect it has on almost all living things at all times. We are almost always in some state of autophagy on the cellular level; however, your cells may not be able to fully engage in the full-blown renewal of the cells that can help prevent disease and slow the aging process. The result of autophagy is that your cells get the deep-clean overhaul that they need to be renewed, refreshed and functioning full steam ahead. And the great thing is that you can activate autophagy through a few, simple steps, but before reading into the activation process, there is more to know about the various types of autophagy. In short, your healthy cells are actively autophagic, and your unhealthy cells are not.

Ch 1.2: Variations of Autophagy

Autophagy was originally noticed by Keith Porter and his student Thomas Ashford in January of 1962. Their reports showed an increased number of lysosomes in rat liver cells after the addition of glucagon. Some of the rats also showed displaced lysosomes near the center of the cell. Originally, they called this discovery autolysis. Unfortunately, Porter and Ashford wrongly interpreted the findings of their experiments as lysosome formation.

Shortly after in 1963, another group of scientists published a detailed description of what they called "focal cytoplasmic degradation," referencing a 1955 German study. The findings detailed three continuous stages of maturation of the cytoplasm to lysosomes. The process was thought to be limited to injury states that functioned under physiological conditions, leading to a rejuvenation of materials and disposal of wasted organelles.

Christian de Duve, a Belgian biochemist, was inspired by the research and decided to call it "autophagy," the Greek word for self-eating. He came up with the name as a part of the lysosomal function while explaining the role of glucagon as a major activator of cell degradation in the liver. He posited that lysosomes are responsible for autophagy. This was the first time that lysosomes were considered the site of intracellular autophagy.

Fast forward to the 1990s when several different groups of scientists discovered autophagy-related genes, independently of each other using the yeast growth for the experiments. Yoshinori Ohsumi and Michael Thumm examined starvation-induced non-selective autophagy, which led to a Pulitzer Prize for Ohsumi and his work in this subject. Another scientist, Daniel Klionsky uncovered the cytoplasm-to-vacuole targeting pathway, a form of selective autophagy. Eventually, they discovered that they were looking at the same pathway from different perspectives. The genes discovered by the yeast experiment groups were given a variety of names like APG, AUT, CVT, GSA, PAG, PAZ, and PDD. A unified name was decided by researchers, using ATG to denote autophagy genes. The 2016 Nobel Prize in Physiology or Medicine was awarded to Yoshinori Ohsumi for these findings.

There has been accelerated growth in the study of autophagy since the early 2000s. Knowledge of ATG genes offered scientists better tools to understand the functions of autophagy in human health and disease. Autophagy and cancer were being closely studied, and there were landmark discoveries within certain research groups showing evidence of the cancer prevention quality of autophagy. Research in neurodegenerative health and auto-immune disease began to take off at this time as well. Since the blossoming of knowledge surrounding autophagy, the studies have continued to gain momentum, and evidence of its ability to heal is still being studied and researched as more and more people bring it into their daily health practices.

There are three main types of autophagy to know, and each one paints a more colorful picture about what is actually happening inside the cell. The three types are macro-autophagy, micro-autophagy, and chaperone-mediated autophagy.

Macro-autophagy

The cell is like a tiny city, comprised of various structures that are all whirring and wheeling to accomplish their inputs and outputs. An autophagosome is a membrane or vesicle in the cell that will fuse with lysosomes.

Autophagosomes form through a process by which omegasomes on the endoplasmic reticulum elongate and become phagophores. Through a communication on the cellular level through the genes Atg 12-Atg-5 and some other chemical complexes, the autophagosome forms and begins to evolve into a spherical shape, encapsulating any free-floating waste, carting it to the lysosome. Imagine Pac Man devouring power pellets. Once the waste material is fully enclosed in the newly formed autophagosome, it will make its way to the nearest lysosome in the cell.

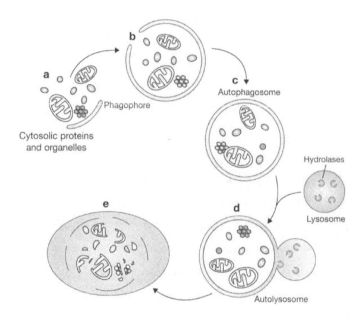

As the recycling plant, the lysosome is full of enzymes to transform waste matter into useful matter. The autophagosome makes contact with the membrane of the lysosome, and they fuse together, allowing the autophagosome to transfer the collected garbage to the recycling plant. Essentially, the autophagosome is the trash collector bringing a truckload of plastic and cardboard to the lysosome to get turned into useful materials.

Micro-autophagy

This process of autophagy is strikingly similar to macro-autophagy, the difference being that the lysosome does all the work. The waste materials are collected like Pac Man chomping pellets; however, in micro-autophagy, the lysosome does the encapsulating and eating. This organelle has the ability to receive waste from the passing autophagosome but can just as easily absorb the waste on its own, meaning that it works twice as hard to clean the cell of unnecessary debris.

The same process of transmutation occurs within the lysosome as it would in macro-autophagy, recycling matter for renewed used and better cell function.

Chaperone-mediated Autophagy (CMA)

With this type of autophagy, the process is much more selective. Unlike macro- and micro-autophagy in which the garbage man just goes around collecting trash, in CMA, there are specific orders and coordinates. It is a timed transfer or translocation of certain protein compounds that need extraction from their current location and guidance by a "chaperone" to the lysosome. CMA is more like a private army who receives orders that must be carried out.

Once you are able to identify the process by understanding the different ways autophagy can occur inside the cell, you can picture the process and connect the dots with why you might want to activate autophagy in your body. If you have never fasted, experienced ketosis through your food intake, or had any kind of exercise routine, then you are likely walking around with some very cluttered cells that need some serious cleanup. Autophagy is always happening on some level; however, when you are not creating circumstances to help it occur optimally, then it is only working at a moderate to low level of efficiency.

There are many ways that initiating autophagy can improve your health and prevent serious or chronic health conditions later in life.

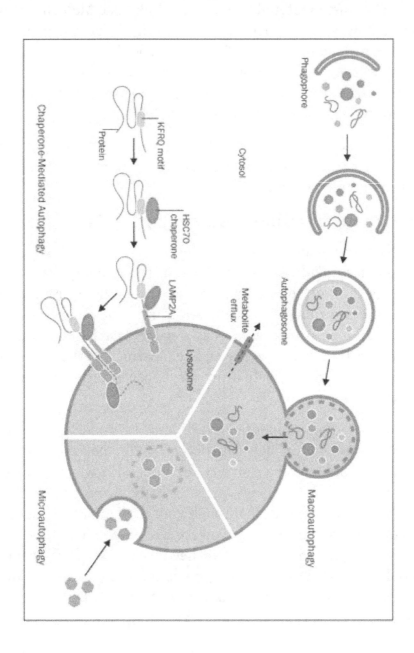

Ch 1.3: Benefits on the Cells, Body, and More

It is the preservation of life when the body is working to fight off something in times of stress or even starvation. This microscopic performance activates to repair the cells and any damage that could be caused by illness and inflammation. This process can also deplete or starve unwanted intruders from the vital nutrients they need to survive, allowing for their death and renewal.

The benefits of autophagy are limitless and can change your body function deep down on the cellular level. Some benefits are:

- *Promotion of a longer, healthier life through cell regeneration*

- *Helps in weight loss by encouraging healthier metabolism*—Autophagy can help clean and restore the toxic accumulation in the mitochondria, the energy makers of the cell. This is where fat gets burned and Adenosine Triphosphate (ATP) is produced. ATP is the compound that provides certain cellular energy, specifically muscle contraction. Autophagy allows for greater efficiency to boost metabolism and energy stores.

- *Risks of neurodegenerative disease are decreased*— Diseases in the brain take a long time to occur and happen over time with the buildup of misfolded, old, or dysfunctional proteins in or around the brain cells. The chemical compounds linked to the cause of Parkinson's disease, synuclein, is removed through autophagy. Studies suggest that the same may be true in cases of

Alzheimer's, removing the compound amyloid from the brain that is known to be associated with this disease. Another neurodegenerative disease is dementia caused by diabetes. Chronic insulin resistance disallows autophagy from occurring so no clean up can occur within the cell, leaving them in a toxic wasteland of malfunction.

- *Regulation of inflammation*—Autophagy allows inflammation when it is needed to fight off invaders, yet also reduces inflammation when it is the chronic response to over-triggered signals to the cells and the body.

- *Helps fight infectious disease*

- *Improves muscle performance*—Muscles undergo stress during exercise. Microscopic tearing in the fibers of muscles occurs during strenuous activity. The muscle fibers, also made of specific kinds of cells, are repaired through the process of autophagy. Over time, as you build muscle, it will reduce the amount of energy needed to utilize the muscle in general.

- *Prevents the onset of cancer*—Though research is still being done to understand the effects of autophagy on various kinds of cancer, studies have indicated that it can help to prevent cancer from forming. Scientists who have studied the impact of impaired autophagic response in mice see an up-rise of cancer in the mice. To perform the study, the mice involved had their autophagic response mechanism cut off from fully functioning. The result was cancer. The question is, can it work as a treatment for cancer, instead of just preventing it through autophagy? How would inducing autophagy impact other treatments?

More research must be done to understand the impact of induced autophagy in pre-existing cancer treatments like chemotherapy, but it may be that it could have a greater benefit than chemo which can be incredibly damaging to the body if applied long term.

- *Improvement in digestive health*—Autophagy is activated through fasting for short periods intermittently. The break from calorie intake and digestion alone can help your digestive system immensely; everyone needs a break now and then. More to that, while your body is resting from needing to digest, the cells that make up your digestive system and all other systems in your body will be activated to perform autophagy because of the fast, leading to a purification of the cells.

- *Improves the health of the skin*—Damage from sun exposure, toxins in the air, changes in temperature, acute ailments like bruises, scrapes, punctures, and burns may all benefit from the autophagic performance. While you may be constantly replacing cells, autophagy keeps the cells fresh and renewed, giving a glow to the skin.

- *Minimizes cell death or apoptosis*—With autophagy functioning, the cells are constantly being cleaned and rejuvenated; without it, the cells are piling up with waste and eventually struggle to perform well, leading to a programmed death of the cell. When that happens, the cell leaves behind trash that needs to be taken out, and if the cell itself is dead, autophagy won't occur because the process occurs inside the cell. The body will have to trigger an inflammatory response to clean up the cell death aftermath.

- *Improved cognition, memory, and brain function*—Autophagy enhances neuroplasticity, the brain's ability to form and reorganize synaptic connections. There is an increase in cognitive ability through the increase of mitochondria. When your brain cells can function well, so can your whole brain.

- *Regulation of hormones, which allows for overall body high performance and function.*

- *Improves cardiovascular health*—Autophagy works to clean toxins and biowaste from the cells of the heart muscle, which is constantly pumping blood through your whole body. Aiding in the general renewal of these cells brings about a better functioning heart.

The list goes on, and discoveries about the effects of autophagy on the health of the body continue to demonstrate the beneficial impact of the autophagic performance. When you create opportunities to enhance and promote autophagy, you are enhancing and promoting the health of every cell in your body.

Ch 1.4: Risks and Cautions of Performance Autophagy

Before you move ahead and begin the process of activating autophagy, it is important to be aware of cautions and risks. To have the best benefit from creating this healing response, you need to plan ahead and be informed about how to do it properly so that you don't cause yourself harm.

There are three main ways that you will learn to activate autophagy in this book: exercise, ketosis, and fasting. When covering the risks, you will understand what can happen or potentially go wrong while using these methods to activate autophagy. Bear in mind that if you are suffering from any severe medical issues, chronic illness, or disease, then it is always a good idea to consult a doctor before beginning this process.

This chapter will briefly cover some of the risks and precautions in initiating autophagy so that you can be prepared to plan your experience well. The next chapters in the book will go into greater detail about each method of activating autophagy.

Some risks and precautions:

- *Losing the wrong kind of weight*—If you lose muscle instead of fat, you are losing the wrong kind of weight. If you don't need to lose a lot of fat through diet, or fasting, then you have to ensure that you consume enough fat prior to fasting. Your body must be prepared to enter a period without calorie intake, and if you have no fat to burn, then you may find yourself losing some muscle. This is not usually the case if you are fasting properly, preparing in advance, and giving your body time to rest while you are on the fast. Some people will try to do intense exercise on a fast to create an even greater increase in the autophagic response. This is when your body will start to turn to the protein of your body for energy. Make sure you are approaching fasting to induce autophagy healthily.

- *Dehydration*—During an intermittent water fast, you may run the risk of dehydration. Fasting is taking a break from food and food contains a percentage of your daily water intake. You will need to make sure you are drinking the right amount of water to stay hydrated. On the other hand, drinking too much water can drown the cells, and drinking too much, too fast can lead to hyponatremia which is the loss of sodium in the body. Loss of salt in your body can lead to an extreme drop in blood pressure. Drop in sodium levels due to excess water will cause fluid shifts from outside to inside the cell. The swell causes pressure in the skull which can lead to headache, nausea, and vomiting. Severe cases of decreased blood pressure can lead to confusion, problems breathing, sleepiness, confused state, weakened muscles, and cramping.

- *Urge to overeat after fasting*—Returning to food after a fast must be done slowly, in steps. When you are not healthily performing a fast, you may be inclined to overeat following the fasting period. If done regularly, this can have a detrimental impact on the body, causing shock to your system.

- *Extreme fasting can lead to starvation and eventually death*

- *If you fast for too long your body will start to eat itself—* If you are performing a fast for an extreme length of time without any calories, or supplements, your body will start to eat muscle, including cardiovascular muscle and also cells like brain cells. This can be avoided by choosing the right length of time for your fast, the right fast for your needs, and the right mineral and vitamin supplement to aid the process and prevent muscle loss. There is an important window of benefit for creating autophagy in a fast—between activation and the point where your body stops burning fat and starts eating muscle.

- *Loss of vitamins and minerals from food can cause health problems*—It is important to allow a mineral supplement. Since there are no calories in many supplements, you will not be breaking the fast, although some vitamins can cause discomfort in the stomach if not taken with food, so finding the right vitamins is important for fasting comfort.

- *Less serious, but important precautions and risks is the effect on mood*—Irritability, moodiness, highs and lows, energy depletion, low blood pressure, and dizziness.

- *Improper fasting can raise stress hormone levels*- If you are not engaging in fasting properly, you may encounter the issue of increased stress hormones in the body which isn't good for long periods, and can be very damaging to many systems.

- *Fast detoxifying can impact your health*—The rate of detox when fasting is rapid. Toxins held in your body fat for long periods will release in your bloodstream as your body burns fat for calorie consumption. Too many toxins in the bloodstream can feel terrible and lead to nausea, sickness, and a general unwell feeling.

- *A fasting high can impact your cognitive ability—* Sometimes during a fast, you may experience fasting high, a feeling of euphoria as your body shifts and heals. Sometimes, this mental state can make it challenging for you to reasonably listen to your body, making sure you are not overdoing it.

A majority of the risks and precautions can be easily avoided if you approach autophagic performance with knowledge and preparation. Because the benefits of autophagy are so powerful, it is worth experiencing. With the right diet, exercise, fasting, and rest, you can healthfully activate autophagy safely and beneficially.

Ch 1.5: Detoxing: The Side Effects

Detoxing is simply your body's process for eliminating toxins. Unlike autophagy which works on the cellular level to eat wastes and toxins to turn them into something better, detoxing requires removal through the bloodstream, skin (sweat, rashes, outbreaks) and excrement or urine. Detoxing can occur through switching to certain diets, specifically designed for detox results, fasting, and exercise.

There are many side effects to detoxing which is why taking care to do it gently and responsibly will allow for a healthier experience overall. Some of the symptoms of detoxing are:

- Skin breakouts in various places

- Body aches and spasms

- Digestive issues (flatulence, bloating, constipation, diarrhea)

- Mood swings

- Mental fog, low cognitive function

- Headache

- Crankiness and irritability

- Flu-like feeling

- Sleep issues

Inflammation from toxins in your body is what causes the symptoms as they are being released. Two to three days of discomfort can occur, depending on the individual, and especially if you are not accustomed to detoxing or have never done it before. Once symptoms clear, there is a feeling of mental clarity, energy, and renewal.

Important, Helpful Guidelines During a Detox

As you eliminate toxins by removing foods slowly into a fasting period, you can support and ease the transition in your body by following these steps:

- Coordinate your primary detox during a time when you can rest, like a weekend, holiday, or scheduled time when you are not working or have any major social plans.

- Eat healthy fats to support your transition and prevent extreme cravings, headaches, and fatigue.

- Drink extra water to help flush toxins from the system.

- Use sweating as well as water consumption to help eliminate toxins through the skin (steam shower, sauna, hot bath).

- Include fiber in your detox diet to eliminate smoothly and avoid constipation.

- Supplement with vitamins and minerals to support muscles, bones, joints, and tissues to prevent achiness, such as magnesium.

- Exercise to help activate detox through blood flow and sweating.

- Get plenty of rest and sleep.

- Include protein in your diet to keep blood sugar balanced (fish, beans, lean poultry, nuts, and seeds).

Symptoms and side effects of detoxing are a good sign that your body is working to eliminate the toxins you are carrying around. Treat yourself well, so you can get to the fasting stage that allows autophagy to work on the cellular level to help detoxify the cells, throughout the entire body.

Chapter 2: Activating Autophagy

This book isn't just about autophagy and what it is from a scientific or biological perspective. The purpose of this book is to show you how you can gain awareness of your own body intelligence to activate the power of your healing ability. It is amazing that we all carry this wisdom deep within our cells, yet most people have no knowledge of this process or why it is important to create opportunities for increased autophagy.

Once you understand the methods for activating autophagy, it is easy to consider bringing it into the fold of your regular diet, exercise, and lifestyle. If you have the knowledge to heal yourself, what would stop you?

So many people are surprised at the idea that we have the mechanisms to prevent and heal our illnesses and diseases. How we have spent the past hundred years, or so, is a direct link to the areas of our history that need attention. Not all science is fact. Some research has come and gone, having been disproven by new discoveries. We see it as a line in the sand when a group of researchers determine something new about long-held wisdom in the medical community. Crossing into the health lines of all, the research shows that one thing hasn't changed in our history as human beings, and that is our cellular design.

The basis of our survival across centuries hasn't come from the fad diet or the present-day version of correct exercise; we all have the understanding deep within us to prevent disease, and yet we can't help but struggle with the reality that men and women across the world are suffering from diseases. If you consider the ancient civilizations of men and women who foraged and hunted, you see that there wasn't any evidence of these illnesses. People might have had incurable ailments or severe injuries that caused an early death; however, cancer was not something detected in any archeological findings of human remains.

Piecing together the common denominators, what do we find? Serious illness isn't all inside us; it comes from everywhere outside of us—our choice of hamburgers and frozen pizza over kale and apples, our addiction to over-the-counter medications that only help you endure the symptoms but not cure the cause, our desire to relax on the couch with a TV show and stay inside with our cell phones, rather than go out for an evening stroll and enjoy the weather. All of these factors are outside of our bodies, and we are the one deciding to create these serious illnesses.

Facing the reality that you are causing your own illness isn't easy for anyone, and letting go of the sugar addictions, coffee habits, and favorite snack foods between meals has its challenges when your body is used to being fed these chemicals regularly.

What you can do to heal yourself is easy; all it takes is an eagerness to try. Because we have the internal body intelligence to heal, we need to know how to allow for that healing to begin. Thanks to the benefits of creating autophagy in our cells, we can now see what it is that is really kicking us into a position of cleansing and renewal.

There are several ways to activate this self-eating/self-healing process. A few of them all together prove to be most beneficial, allowing for a balanced, autophagic occurrence. When you start to ignite the process, you will understand the connection between each method of activation and how the healthier approach to stabilizing an autophagic detox will utilize several ways together. Like the cogs and wheels all working together to tell time.

Understanding each method separately will allow for a more fine-tuned, intentional approach to autophagy. It is important when activating this method of deep cellular healing that you attend to it carefully and healthily. Electing to use each method during your intentional autophagic activation, will provide you with the best results for internal repair and deep healing.

This chapter will approach each method and explain the how and why of each method as a source of autophagic initiation. Further chapters in this book will give more step by step guidance on performing these methods for increased autophagy.

Ch 2.1: Ways to Initiate Autophagy

There are multiple ways by which autophagy is activated in both plants and animals that occur in the natural world without design or purposeful initiation. When your body is operating optimally, autophagy is occurring optimally also. In our current culture, the air we breathe, the water we drink, the multiple meals a day full of carbs, sugars, stimulants, and highly processed materials default our bodies to a setting of low performance. The elegant autophagic dance within cannot occur properly under such conditions, and in order to return to balanced levels of regularly occurring autophagy in our cells, we must begin by initiating the process and using the methods of activation to assist our bodies in healthy cell regeneration.

Before you get started with preparing to activate autophagy intentionally, it is important to understand how and why the methods outlined in this chapter work to promote that process. The major methods that will be discussed and detailed in this chapter are exercise, ketosis fasting, and intermittent water fasting.

Exercise

The benefits of exercise are long proven to establish a healthy, balanced body. The effects of exercise on all systems of the body are profound, and autophagy is part of the reason for this. The stress you put on your muscles when you exercise brings about the activation of autophagy. There are a variety of ways to exercise, and some of them create a deeper impact on the cellular level than others. Exercise is also a large part of a smooth detoxification process. When you exercise, you increase your heart rate which pushes more fresh, oxygenated blood at a faster rate through your body, allowing for a swifter push and release of toxins coming out through a fasting or detox process, kind of like flushing the toilet.

With certain kinds of exercise, you can create a more impactful autophagic response, and coupled with some of the other methods, you bring about greater change and more abundant cell regeneration, upwards of 300% from if you weren't exercising at all, according to some research.

Ketosis

The process by which the body relies on fat stores for energy rather than sugars and carbohydrates is known as ketosis. More specifically, when certain foods are eliminated from the diet, the body turns to stored fats to burn as fuel. When the fat is used as energy, acids are left behind in the blood and are eliminated in the urine. These acids are known as ketones and are the indicator that you need to assure that fat is being burned.

Restricting calories in the diet and eliminating certain foods such as carbohydrates and sugars that turn into glucose, can stimulate the autophagic process by bringing about the change in cells through diet and ketosis.

Fasting

Fasting hasn't lost its mainstream impact since the dawn of early humans who scavenged the Earth for food. As we evolve, we can connect the dots more and more about certain methods of health and healing and the correlation with our early ancestors. Refraining from and restricting certain foods and eliminating them altogether, create an internal survival gateway to boost your body's need to stay alive until your next meal.

This connection to autophagy is what truly eliminates the wastes and toxins. As your diet becomes less involved, fewer meals and longer time between them, you instigate the action of cell renewal throughout the body systems. When you disengage from food for fuel, your body can rely on fat for fuel and give your cells an opportunity to clean house, so to speak.

Positive performance autophagy requires initiation through some food elimination and fasting. There are healthy methods and approaches as well as risks and dangers, so it will be important to have a handle on proper fasting methods before jumping in.

Intermittent Water Fasting

Along the history of humankind's search for food in times of foraging and hunting, at times, the only thing available was water. In today's health news, everyone insists on 8 glasses of water as the essential minimum requirement. The internal essence of every part of you, every muscle, organ, fiber, and cell, is water.

What you gain from fasting from food is an activation of autophagy; the goal of which is to recycle cell waste and rejuvenate the body from the cellular level. What you lose in the fasting process is water. Upwards of 30% of your daily water intake comes from food. When you take food away, you replace it with water. That is the basis of water fasting.

Intermittency is the timing of fasting for healthy, balanced autophagic performance. It will obviously cause irreparable damage to the body if you fast too long, too frequently. Fasting for short term periods is a healthy way to reestablish cellular function, and should be done alternating between eating a healthy diet and igniting autophagy with fasting.

As you can see, each method has its value and purpose in initiating autophagy. Together, these methods bring about cell renewal and regeneration, elimination of toxins, and prevention of disease. In the next sub-chapters, we will dig deeper into each method, assuring that you can healthily support autophagy for healing the cells.

Ch 2.2: Exercise

What happens to your body when you exercise? The answer lies on a deep, cellular level, not just in the physical results. Since early human existence, we have had to adapt and perform using our bodies to leverage the entire experience. Our bones, muscles, and tissues are what support us, keep us upright, and help us handle all activities in our everyday lives. Regardless of whether you are a caveman or a bank teller, you are using your muscles, bones, joints, and tissues, all of which are made up of tiny cells, specifically designed to function for each body process.

Early man had a greater need and opportunity to have regular exercise; it was the only way to survive. Before the advent of automobiles, factories, industry, and technology, human beings were required to use their bodies all the time, every day to accomplish the ins and outs of human existence. An exercise wasn't something you had to plan or schedule. Gym memberships were not a necessary part of reality. Life was exercise unless you were royalty and could lay around all day and eat decadent food to your heart's content, or rather discontent.

To understand the need for exercise on your body, you must look deep within the muscles and understand them on a cellular level. Bringing into focus the structure and function of your muscles, will bring you closer to understanding how autophagy can have an impact on this system, and why you want to create autophagy to heal this part of yourself.

Muscle is considered a soft tissue. It is found in most animals. Muscle cells are made of protein filaments that contain actin and myosin. These protein filaments glide past one another, creating contractions that change the length and the shape of the cell. Think of a bulging bicep: the muscle fibers collectively bulge to produce that shape when a certain action occurs. Force and motion are the functions of muscles. They have many roles such as moving your body in various ways, posture, internal organ movements like a heartbeat, and peristalsis, which is the movement of the digestive organs to move food through the body.

Myogenesis is the process by which the mesodermal layer of embryonic cells creates muscle tissue. The muscles can be divided into three types: striated (skeletal), smooth, and cardiac. The action of the muscle is either voluntary or involuntary. Involuntary muscles do not require conscious thought to function; they just perform their tasks, and you don't even realize it. The beat of the heart in cardiac muscle and the peristalsis of the intestines are examples of involuntary muscle movement. Skeletal or striated muscled requires conscious thought to move and is therefore called voluntary muscle movement. There are fast and slow twitch fibers when talking about skeletal muscle.

Oxidation of fats and carbohydrates is what powers muscles to make them move. Fast twitch fibers in skeletal muscles also use anaerobic chemical reactions. The reactions of the chemicals are what produced ATP, and adenosine triphosphate is what gives energy to the movement of the myosin heads in the muscle fibers.

The epimysium is a layer of tough connective tissue that sheaths the skeletal muscles. This tough tissue is what pins down the muscle tissues to the tendons. Bundles of fascicles lie within the epimysium, each one containing anywhere from 10 to 100 or more muscle fibers, all sheathed by another layer of tissue called perimysium. The perimysium is a pathway for nerves and blood flow to your muscles. Myocytes are the muscle cells and are like bundles of threads, encapsulated in its own collagenous endomysium tissue. The overall muscle is made up of all these tiny fibers that are all bundled together in fascicles to form your muscles. Every muscle is built of muscle cells.

Muscle function is supported by the membranes that surround each bundle, giving the energy and stamina it needs to resist passive stretching and maintain active performance.

Each muscle cell contains myofibrils. These are also bundled protein filaments and are complex strands of a variety of filaments that form to create sarcomeres. Sarcomeres are like candy canes, striated due to the intermittent layout of the skeletal and cardiac muscle. Actin and myosin are the filament components of the sarcomere.

There are significant differences between the three types of muscle, yet they all have the same cell function provided by the actin and myosin. The actin and myosin are what create the contraction of the muscle on the cellular level. The contraction of skeletal muscle on the cellular level is controlled by nerves that send electrical impulses from the brain, specifically, motoneurons (also cells). There are internal, pacemaker cells that are responsible for the involuntary movement of the cardiac and smooth muscles. The chemical neurotransmitter acetylcholine is what facilitates all skeletal and most smooth muscle contraction.

Movement of almost every muscle is decided by the origin and insertion of that muscle: where it comes from and what it attaches to. However, many sarcomeres are able to operate in a cross section of muscle determines the amount of force it can generate; the bigger your muscles, the thicker the sarcomeres, the greater the force. Every skeletal muscle is made of myofibrils, each one a chain of sarcomeres. The muscle cell contracts as one unit of sarcomeres, shortening simultaneously and lengthening simultaneously.

Leverage mechanics determines the amount of force that can occur in the action of the muscles in the external environment. An example of this would be flexing your biceps muscle.

Much of the body's energy consumption is through the movement of your muscles. Every muscle cell produces ATP which is the energy compound that creates the power to move the myosin heads in every muscle fiber. There is a short-term store of energy know as creatine phosphate, and it is born from the ATP. It can also regenerate ATP when it is needed with the compound known as creatine kinase. Muscles will also keep a store of glycogen, which is a form of glucose. It can be quickly turned into glucose when there is a need for sustained energy during incredibly powerful muscle contractions.

The molecule of glucose can be broken down anaerobically during glycolysis. Out of glycolysis 2 ATP and 2 lactic acid molecules are formed; however, this outcome is not produced in the aerobic state. Each muscle cell also has fat molecules that are utilized as energy during aerobic exercise. It takes longer to produce ATP in aerobic energy systems and requires more involved steps, yet it produces a great deal more ATP than what is seen in anaerobic glycolysis.

On another note, cardiac muscle can regularly consume all of the macronutrients listed above: protein, glucose, and fat. It can do this aerobically, as it is always working and pumping blood throughout the body. Also, the cardiac muscle will always take out the maximum amount of ATP from any involved molecule. These muscle fibers, as well as the liver and red blood cells, often consume lactic acid that is usually put out by the skeletal muscles during exercise; in essence, exercise helps the cells of your heart function.

Human muscle efficiency has been measured at up to 18-26%. This ratio comes from a breakdown of the output of mechanical work against the total metabolism, calculated from the consumption of oxygen. Low efficiency comes from a lowered generation of ATP from your food energy intake, and also the loss of converting ATP into mechanical action within the muscle fibers, as well as overall mechanical loss within the body. The loss of efficiency depends on the type of exercise being performed and the type of muscle fibers being used.

Having an understanding of the cellular function of muscles is vital when you are considering the way autophagy works. To break it down, muscle is the result of three, important things:

1. Physiological strength = size of the muscle, cross section of muscle, response to training

2. Neurological strength = the strength of signal given to the muscles telling them to contract (strong or weak signal)

3. Mechanical strength = force, leverage, joint capability

Discovering the lessons within the cells brings you face to face with the commitment, to knowing the inner workings of the cell's ability to not only perform their functions but also their ability to heal. The fine tuning that occurs deep within comes from the sophisticated machinery that makes up your entire being: the cell. Muscle cells are as in need of autophagy as any other part of your body. Your muscles are your body, and if your muscle cells are unable to renew, then you lose the quality of function that keeps you feeling young and agile.

The vitality of out muscle health begins in the cell, like with all other systems in the body. One of the significant ways to activate autophagy is through the exercise of the muscles. Seeing the muscle up close helps you understand what is happening deep within when you exercise. The cells need cleansing so that your body can perform optimally. If you never exercise, how can your muscle cells do the work they are intended to do?

As we have engineered ways to unload the burden of labor onto machines and technology, we have accrued a need to find our daily dose of exercise in other ways. Many people have given up on exercise altogether, living in a culture that promotes a sedentary lifestyle in front of a TV, or a need to work for 8 hours straight sitting at a computer.

Our bodies need exercise to function well, and this has been proven over and over again. Benefits of exercise are far-reaching and here are a few examples:

- *Good for muscles and bones*—building and maintenance and the release of hormones to absorb amino acids in muscle and bone.

- *Increased energy levels*

- *Reduced risk of chronic disease*—improved insulin use, reduction of belly fat which leads to Type II diabetes, improved cardiovascular health, hormonal balance, oxygen-rich blood to improve the vital function of all body systems.

- *Weight loss*—there are three ways to lose weight: digestion, body functions like breathing and heartbeat, and exercise. Exercise increases your metabolism and when combined with the right diet promotes weight loss.

- *Improved brain health, memory and cognitive function*—hormonal stimulation as well as oxygen-rich blood help the brain function optimally.

- *Improved skin health*—Your integumentary system is your largest organ and is an organ of elimination. Releasing toxins through the skin from exercise and sweating, can have a profound impact on the overall health of the skin.

- *Pain reduction*—Exercise provides a regulation of all body systems, enhancing the performance of cellular function allowing for the release and regulation of inflammation in the body which causes pain.

- *Sleep regulation*—regular exercise has been proven to aid your ability to sleep well. Physical exertion gives your body the opportunity to burn the energy in your body from all of the food you ate throughout the day. If you do not exercise and continue to consume calories, your body will want to burn the caloric energy in some way, keeping you awake or restless through the night so that the energy can be burned.

- *Improved mood*—Exercise releases serotonin in the brain which is the happy hormone. Your mood will feel more uplifted and happier as a result of exercise.

The one completely overlooked aspect of all the benefits of exercise is that autophagy links to each benefit, causing the outcome to occur. What we feel or see on the outside as increased energy, happier mood, healthier body, and better sleep is the direct result of autophagy.

Every single cell in your body is contacted during the exercise experience. When you look at all of the cells operating as a whole universe of information and regulation, you can see how exercise can benefit not only the muscles and bones but every activity and function of the human body brought out by the action of autophagy. Exercise increases positive stress levels in the body. The act of engaging the muscles, skeleton, joints, ligaments, and tissues through specific motions causes fatigue in the fibers and even microscopic tearing. Even further in depth, the tears ask for repair through the sophistication of the cellular system, activating and increasing autophagy.

You certainly can create an autophagic response in the cells without exercise; however, for a balanced and healthy experience of healing the body, exercise will always be of benefit to you. Variations on the kinds of exercise and levels of intensity are encouraged and recommended. Overuse of any muscle group or excessive weight lifting can also cause internal damage. It is a fine line to walk, so make sure you know what you are doing before you hurt yourself with exercise. Finding a balance with exercise styles will help improve and regulate autophagy, especially in combination with the other methods for activating this process.

Ch 2.3: Ketosis

Caloric intake in our early days as humans was highly limited. Agriculture wasn't invented yet and people hunted and gathered to survive, covering large distances regularly and fasting between meals. Typical diets were plants, seeds, nuts, fruits, and occasionally meats that were successfully hunted. Animal protein and fat were like drinking at an oasis after a long journey through the desert; it was what the body was ready for after a low calorie to no calorie intake and would replenish the body for more long distances ahead.

Ketosis is the metabolic state where some of the body's energy supply comes from ketones in the blood, rather than a state of glycolysis (glucose in the blood provides the energy). Ketosis will occur when the body is metabolizing fat quickly and converting fatty acids into ketones. It's a nutritional process distinguished by serum concentrations of ketone bodies with normal levels of insulin and blood glucose. Ketogenesis is the formation of ketone bodies that occurs when liver glycogen stores are exhausted, and sometimes from metabolizing MCT or medium chain triglycerides. There are also ketone supplements that you can consume along with your other daily vitamins.

The levels of ketone bodies are regulated mostly by insulin and glucagon. A majority of cells in the body can use both glucose and ketone bodies for fuel. During ketosis, cells can also use free fatty acids and glucose synthesis.

Long-term ketosis can be the result of fasting or keto-diets. Deliberately inducing ketosis serves as a medical intervention for a variety of conditions. During glycolysis, high levels of insulin encourage the storage of body fat and block its release from adipose tissues. In ketosis, fat reserves are readily released and consumed.

There are two sources of ketone bodies: fatty acids in adipose tissue and ketogenic amino acids.

Your adipose tissue can be relied on to store fatty acids which allow for the regulation of temperature and energy in the body. Fatty acids can be released by adipokine, a cell signaling protein, alerting the body to high glucagon and levels of epinephrine, an inverse correspondence to low insulin levels. High glucagon and low insulin relate to times of fasting and also to times when blood glucose levels are low. Fatty acids are metabolized in the mitochondria of the cell in order to produce energy; however, free fatty acids are unable to penetrate cellular membranes due to their negative electrical charge. This leads to an enzyme bond: coenzyme A is bound to the fatty acid to produce acyl-CoA and can now enter the mitochondria.

Now inside the mitochondria, the bound fatty acids are used as fuel in the cells through oxidation, which cuts two carbons off of the acyl-CoA molecule to form a new compound, acetyl-CoA. This new substance enters a citric acid cycle. Citric acid then enters the tricarboxylic acid which creates a very high energy yield in the original fatty acid.

Ketone bodies are also produced in mitochondria and are the response to low blood glucose levels.

During ketogenesis, two acetyl-CoA molecules condense to form acetoacetyl-CoA via thiolase, an enzyme. Acetoacetyl-CoA combines with another acetyl-CoA to form the ketone body acetoacetate. Ketone bodies can be exported from the liver to supply crucial energy to the brain when blood glucose levels are low.

So, what does all of this mean? To break it down simply, ketosis occurs on the cellular level when you are low on glycogen in the body due to a lack of calories or a low carbohydrate diet. Your body burns fat through a sophisticated response and call of the chemicals in your cells. Everything is about balance on the microscopic level.

Ketosis is in balance when the body can burn stored fats. If the body has no fat reserves, or there is no fat being ingested, the body will feed on the proteins or muscles. When your body's insulin is not effectively utilized due to damaged, fatigued and dirty cell waste, ketones can accrue in the body creating a highly acidic internal landscape that can lead to illness and sometimes chronic disease. High acid inside the body is detrimental long term and requires a more balanced pH through the foods you eat, how much water you drink, and your vitamin and mineral intake.

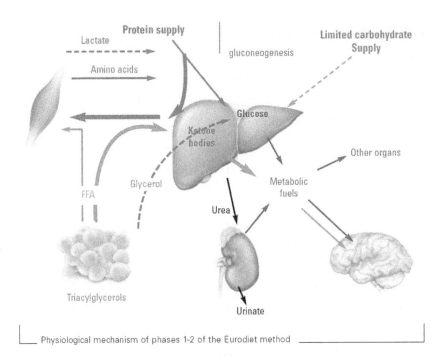

Physiological mechanism of phases 1-2 of the Eurodiet method

High acid from ketones is known as ketoacidosis and is most often seen in people with diabetes who have issues with insulin regulation. It can also occur in extreme athletes who are overexerting their bodies over long periods with no caloric intake. Think of a triathlete trying to make it to the end of the race after the intensity of the exercises with little to no food. They can also experience ketoacidosis. Another example is childbirth. If a mother is laboring for days without eating, her body can start to react in this way.

Insulin and Ketosis

It is important to understand the role of insulin in ketosis. Insulin is produced in the pancreas, and it is energy, pure energy. Your body's cells use it to regulate proper intake of sugars in the body to operate efficiently. If your cells cannot receive proper doses of insulin, it will be rejected by the cell and end up in the bloodstream. Hyperglycemia is often a result of insulin production that can't release into the cells which chronically occurs and turns into diabetes.

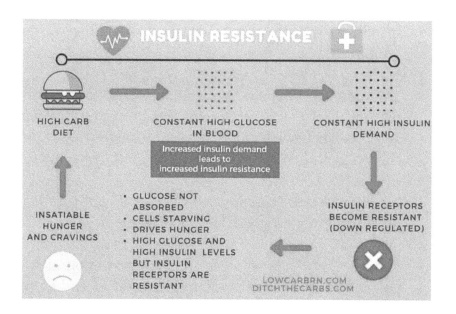

What happens when your insulin production and intake are not effective or functional, is that your energy stores cannot regulate either. And the release of insulin in the blood creates acid or ketones, that lead to an overactive state of ketosis in which you are no longer burning fat. The body holds the fat, keeping you overweight, and starts to lock onto proteins, like the muscle. The exit of ketones from your body occurs through urination, and when you get tested for levels of ketones, it is your body's alert system that you are experiencing functional or dysfunctional insulin uptake due to a chronic overabundance of sugar in the blood. Your body doesn't know how to handle this, so systems begin to malfunction on a deep cellular level.

Here are some important facts you should know regarding insulin:

- Insulin resistance increases your risk of getting diabetes.

- You might be insulin resistant for years and not even know it.

- Insulin resistance usually doesn't trigger any obvious symptoms.

- The American Diabetes Association (ADA) has suggested that up to fifty percent of people with insulin resistance and prediabetes will develop type 2 diabetes if they don't change their diet, exercise, and other lifestyle factors.

- Insulin resistance can increase the risk of obesity or being overweight, high triglycerides, high blood pressure.

- Insulin resistance may develop a skin condition in some people known as acanthosis nigricans. It looks like soft, dark patches sometimes on the back of the neck and armpits.

- A buildup of insulin within skin cells can cause acanthosis nigricans.

You may not be anywhere close to having diabetes; however, insulin resistance over time can lead to prediabetes and eventually type 2 diabetes. Seeing a doctor is the best option, and autophagy can be an added aid in preventing insulin resistance, that leads to diabetes and turning current diabetes around for the better.

Diabetes symptoms:

- Extreme thirst or hunger

- Having hunger, even after having just eaten

- Increased and/or frequent urination

- Tingling sensations in hands or feet

- Excessive fatigue

- Having infections often

There are tests you can take to test your blood sugar levels to find out if you are insulin resistant. The A1C test is the test given by a doctor to help measure your average blood sugar. It may be useful to get tested, so you have an idea of how autophagy can help you become less insulin resistant.

The test measurements look something like this:

- An A1C under 5.7 percent = normal.

- An A1C between 5.7 and 6.4 percent = prediabetes diagnoses.

- An A1C equal to or above 6.5 percent = diabetes diagnoses.

You can also have a fasting blood glucose test which shows your fasting blood sugar level. This test is done after not eating or drinking for at least eight hours.

- Fasting blood sugar levels under 100 milligrams/deciliter (mg/dL) = normal.

- Levels between 100 and 125 mg/dL = prediabetes diagnoses.

- Levels equal to or greater than 126 mg/dL = diabetes.

A glucose tolerance test is another way to diagnose prediabetes or diabetes. Your blood glucose level is determined before this test begins, after which you receive a premeasured sugary drink. Your blood glucose level is then checked again 2 hours later.

- Blood sugar level after two hours of less than 140 mg/dL = normal.

- Result between 140 mg/dL and 199 mg = prediabetes.

- Blood sugar level of 200 mg/dL or higher = diabetes.

According to the American Diabetes Association, if you have insulin resistance, you may prevent diabetes by exercising 30 minutes, 5 days a week and eating a balanced diet. Losing weight can lower your risk of developing diabetes. Imagine what miracles you could work by activating autophagy.

Autophagy is the cleaning crew reaction that begins the change to reorganize cells for better insulin absorption. Without our insulin, the body's sugar levels would derail, and we would only eat off of our tissues. Thankfully, we all have insulin production coming from the pancreas, and can benefit the body by understanding how insulin works and how to regulate our diet and exercise, to allow for proper insulin sensitivity. For autophagy to correct this insulin dysfunction allowing for proper ketogenic performance, a resistance to foods can cause an internal turn of events that allows for proper cell function, namely cell clean-up.

Letting the cells control the dynamic inner world brings about the best body performance. Focusing energy inside the cell, autophagy consumes a great build-up of waste materials that causes the insulin resistance that leads to detrimental disease, and possible ketoacidosis.

What you want from ketosis is a healthy burning of fat fuel. When you are relying on fat stores, you can maintain healthy weight loss and weight consistency. Ketosis is promoted through autophagy, and in order to allow for healthy ketosis, a certain diet must be applied and practiced allowing for fat burning and toxin release.

Complex carbohydrates and sugars are eliminated to renew proper insulin use, performance autophagy, and ketosis. Testing ketosis is a way you can observe if you have activated autophagy in your cells. You can purchase Ketone Strips that change color when applied to urine samples and demonstrate ketone levels in the body, ranging from no ketosis to healthy ketosis to ketoacidosis.

Engaging in the benefits of ketosis will help your body properly produce and utilize insulin, and use fat stores for fuel which assists in healthy weight loss without losing muscle.

Ch 2.4: Fasting

What you don't eat won't kill you, but extensive fasting will starve you to death. There is a fine line to walk regarding fasting to encourage autophagy, and damaging your lifeline connected to food. In reality, no wonder drug can cause an autophagic response in the body. The only way to truly enact the self-eating mechanism of the cell is to deplete the energy in the body by eliminating food.

Your energy is stored in each and every cell inside your system of life. The chemicals produced to create energy in the body release as needed to perform various functions. What if you needed to end the cycle of calories your body receives every day in order to allow for better cell performance?

Fasting gains on autophagy. What this means is that as you reduce the number of calories you ingest in a day you kick start autophagy. While your body is doing less to digest food and circulate nutrients in your body, creating new forms of energy, the cells have a hiatus from exposure to added energy and materials to process and can function to ball up all the garbage and throw it in the recycling bin. It's hard to work in the cell, and most of us aren't thinking microscopically when we eat our daily bread.

Today's diet is extreme. Most Americans eat 3-square meals a day with snacks in between, coffee, sugar, additives, and highly processed foods that are chemically engineered in laboratories, as well as endless quantities of prescription drugs and over the counter medications. On top of all those toxins, the average American is chronically dehydrated, choosing sugary beverages over clean water. There is no way to effectively flush the toxins under those conditions.

What happens when you keep adding calories, limit exercise and refrain from regular water consumption? Disease, obesity, mental and physical stress, mental and physical illness, depression, anxiety, trouble sleeping, inflammation, and more.

When you realize the detrimental impact of the American diet on the cellular level, you begin to understand the chronic disease plaguing the nation. The answer is simple: fasting for autophagic performance.

When people think of fasting, they think of rail-thin, bony people who are making a religious or political sacrifice, like Gandhi or the suffragette, Alice Paul. They think of individuals who succumb to extreme dieting methods to lose weight, no matter the cost and end up with psychological disorders like Anorexia Nervosa and Bulimia.

Fasting for health is not starvation. There are limits to consider when approaching this method for activating autophagy. What you find, rather than severe loss of food intake and extreme measures of weight loss, is a carefully regulated and balanced approach to caloric restriction and food elimination. You do not eliminate it permanently; it is a temporary act to elicit the autophagic response.

Many fasts are only 16-18 hours, several days a week, while others may last 24-72 hours with healthy boundaries of when it is too long. Here are a few fasting methods to consider:

- *Time-restricted*—This will include a daily ratio of time that you are not eating and the time that you are. A common ratio is 16:8 whereby you fast for 16 hours and allow food for 8 out of the full 24-hour day. You can adjust the ratio as long as the fasting time is at least 16 hours for a maximum autophagic benefit.

- *Alternate Day Fasting*—Here, you will alternate days you eat with days you don't. Essentially, Monday you eat food; Tuesday you don't. Wednesday you eat food; Thursday you don't, etc.

- *Intermittent Fasting*—This is a full 24+ hour day fast separated by days or weeks. That could look like one day fast once a week or twice a month, or perhaps a 2-3 day fast once a month.

- *5:2 Diet and Fast*—This ratio suggests eating for 5 days and fasting for 2 every week.

- *Low-Calorie Fast*—This kind of fast includes an extreme reduction of calorie intake over a period of time but still allows for some calories to be ingested.

- *Religious or Political Fasting*—This is beyond the scope of this book; however, these kinds of fasts are important to the beliefs of some individuals. It is important that no matter the reason for the fast, you should see to it that you are doing it in a healthy, balanced way.

The basic tactic is to resist food long enough to promote autophagy. Permitting this small fasting time multiple days, a month, or year can reduce your body's cell deterioration significantly.

What you don't want to do, is extend the fast to the point that your body overextends ketosis which causes acidic cell damage, that can lead to fatality and bring about unnecessary starvation, that causes the body to eat muscle rather than fat stores. This is why engaging in short-lived fasting can provide autophagic cell renewal, while burning fat and restoring optimal cell function.

Dieting has been proven to benefit in the short term; however, most people try to tricking their bodies into losing weight without engaging in autophagy and ketosis. While some diets can be useful under certain conditions and for certain ailments, a majority of mainstream diets lead to insulin resistance, weight retention, and problematic sugar highs and lows that lead to binge eating.

Waste in the cells can easily accumulate under these conditions and without autophagic response initiation, the waste will build, the cells will operate at a dysfunctional or slow level, and balanced health will not be fully restored. Fasting improves the body's ability to restore itself. Taking short breaks from food intake has been scientifically proven to activate autophagy, which allows the cells in your body to clean up and reorganize, leading to a fresher, healthier, more youthful you.

In addition to the overall health benefit of food fasting, research is also showing that autophagy induced by fasting, has an impact on the healing of chronic illness and disease. There have been reports that creating this response in the body while battling cancer, diabetes, and inflammatory diseases can allow for deeper, cellular healing and prevention of future recurrence of the illness that cannot be remedied by prescription drugs, chemotherapy, or surgery.

This is your body intelligence at its finest. We are sophisticated machines that have the capability to self-heal, and creating the autophagic process through careful, healthful fasting could very well save your life.

Ch 2.5: Intermittent Water Fasting

Water is life. No cell in your body can function without it. No living thing on Earth can exist without water's vital essence. Because performance autophagy relates to cell tissue cleansing and renewal, without water, this process would be null and void. The basic human cell is protein, fat, cholesterol, and water. While you begin to increase autophagy through fasting and ketosis, you begin the process of reducing wastes and toxins in the body on a cellular level.

Water will get used to performing all these functions, collecting and disposing of exhausted materials and compounds. The point of energy is to give life to our experience. The point of water is to give life to that energy. Because water is so significant to the system as a whole, water fasting is a described method of autophagy on account of its ability to enhance autophagic reaction and response.

Timing is everything. Intermittence is a level of time which allows your body to receive ample energy through healthy eating and diet, followed by moments and periods of fasting. This alternating effect brings about effective autophagy, giving space and time to the cells to renew and for the body to gain nutrients; both are necessary for optimal health.

Water fasting is the method by which all food is eliminated slowly over the course of several hours and/or days to allow your body time to gently respond and react to fewer calories. Water is then increased to allow for proper autophagic response and activity. The only thing consumed in water fast is water; however, some vitamins and minerals may be consumed for proper internal balance. Although no calories are ingested, some vitamins and minerals are necessary for the proper function of the cells so that they may do their work during autophagy.

Water is essential; it carries all life and acts as the conduit of all internal function and performance. Without it, autophagy wouldn't work. Balancing the fast with extra water is key to healthy autophagic response and brings about greater change, renewal and deep cellular healing.

Chapter 3: Autophagy Performance

The answer to autophagy is in the question of how you want to look at your own health and healing. Too many people are trying to perform at the same level using the same tricks of the trade, flopping back and forth between all of the culturally popular diet crazes, and falling off the wagon on account of highs, lows, and cravings. If you understand how autophagy works, then you also understand that to look at it from the point of view of universal success isn't going to work.

Yes, all of our cells have the same function of cell renewal and autophagy, but no one has the same genetic make-up, DNA, and body type. We can't all fit into the same box, which is why you need to resist the tendency to adopt the program that everyone else is using. We don't have the same reasons for going on diets, exercising, and looking for the cure to health problems. From an outside point of view, it can look the same: weight loss, bigger muscles, long life. However, tapping into the reality of autophagy means truly looking at and listening to your body wisdom.

You are going to heal under the right circumstances for you, but what are those conditions? You can't take the exact same routine from your neighbor and expect the same results; it just doesn't work that way. In order to see a true turn around in your health, you have to tinker with the plan for healing that is unique to you.

Following the instructions of any diet, weight loss, and exercise program can feel like a lot of work. When you fall, of course, there can be a lot of doubt and discouragement that leads to continuing old patterns of eating and digesting. What you get out of autophagy is so much more than the common weight loss program, because it isn't just about weight loss and muscle building; it's about deep cellular healing for long lasting life.

Because our culture stresses all of the weight loss routines and breaking bad habits, we find ourselves pigeon-holed into dieting in short-lived spurts for short term effect, rather than altering the concept of our internal workings and changing our bodies from deep within on the microscopic level. It isn't just how you look on the outside; it's how you feel deep within and how your cells perform and function.

Creating autophagy for health benefits isn't hard. It's not a gimmick or a fad; it's your body intelligence working for you behind the scenes, and all you have to do is create the right conditions for that to occur. You may find some general theories and practices in this book that can help you get started with your renewal program; however, so much of the experience is going to be your own awareness of how your body works and how it doesn't. Your heredity can play a big part in your body structure and body top, meaning that not everyone will look the same when they lose 30 pounds.

Our anatomy is based on the same principles of structure and function that clean and heal us constantly, without obvious notice, but if we are not doing the work to create those circumstances, how can we put that gift to the test? Bringing autophagy to the foreground in your food intake, fasting and exercise cycles can change your whole health and reality.

This chapter will go into greater detail what you can do specifically to enact autophagy through guidelines and steps to understanding each diet, fast and muscle performance so you can fine-tune the healing experience that is right for you.

Ch 3.1: Ketosis Diets

Weight loss occurs for every one differently. We all have our genetic background, healthy or unhealthy eating habits and a long list of favorite snacks and treats that we go, for when we need an exciting pick-me-up. On the day to day level, we pick and graze between meals and have an endless number of options to choose from at the grocery store and restaurants. Many of us enjoy a large quantity of carbohydrates, delicious sugary food and drink, and a hearty helping of premade convenience foods regularly.

All of these factors, from the dietary standpoint, are what lead to the internal cell deficiency that autophagy works to heal. Because we all have our unique internal make-up, it is important to listen to our bodies when beginning to shift into ketosis diets, or keto-diets, as they are often called.

There are side effects of starting ketosis that can cause flu-like feelings that will discourage continuation of the diet. Often times, these symptoms are the result of changing too much, too soon and can be prevented by gently easing into a change in diet, rather than going from zero to 100 mph.

What you can do is slowly start eliminating certain foods one day at a time to control your body's release of toxins. This tactic is known as partial-elimination of these problematic foods. Ranging from days to weeks, careful elimination of these foods will lead to a healthier experience when adopting a new eating plan. Slow adaptation to this new diet will have fewer unpleasant side effects when approached in this way.

Most ketosis diets are relatively similar, but there are a few to consider when looking to create autophagy. They are:

- *Standard Keto Diet (75-20-5)*—This diet involves a ratio of fat to protein to carbohydrates, like the other keto diets will; however, the ratio in this diet usually creates the most noticeable change in the body resulting from fat loss and has a more profound impact overall on activating autophagy. The ratio is 75 percent fat, 20 percent protein, and 5 percent carbohydrates (75-20-5 daily intake). Keep in mind that based on your BMI, or body mass index, the measurements for these amounts will be different from person to person. If you weigh 160 lbs., versus someone who weighs 260, you will need to account for some change in measurement regarding the quantity of food, keeping the overall percentage of daily intake the same.

- *High Protein Keto Diet (60-35-5)*—This diet is similar to the standard keto diet, the only difference being the ratio shift. Rather than consuming 75 percent fat, it drops down to 60 percent, allowing for a higher percentage of protein daily. The reason someone might choose this ratio is if they are working to promote more muscle building rather than fat loss. For some people, starting with the standard diet helps them shave off the fat pounds, and once they have reached that goal they continue the keto diet, shifting to a high protein diet to help build muscle, especially if there isn't a large quantity of fat stores to burn.

- *Cyclical Keto Diet (5:2)*—Like with a 5:2 fasting ratio, this keto diet applies a method for exchanging fats for carbs on a 5 to 2 basis. For the first five days, you will eat a standard ketosis diet. For the following two days, you switch the ratio so that instead of high fat you are eating high carb (70-75% carb, 20-25% protein, 5-10% fat). This diet is often utilized for high-performance athletes who need a major carb load for weightlifting or workouts. It helps to create a balanced fat loss while building muscle mass.

- *Targeted Keto Diet (carbs before exercise)*—This diet is like a hybrid diet of the standard and the cyclical keto diets. You maintain a typical standard keto diet and digest your daily carb allotment half an hour before your workout, allowing for muscle building and stamina in the workout without taking time off of ketosis.

For the best results for autophagy performance, the standard and high protein diets are the best choices for creating ketosis and initiating an autophagic response. The other two diets may be more beneficial on a long-term track and should be considered, especially if you are a bodybuilder or athlete that requires more carb intake for building muscle and using energy.

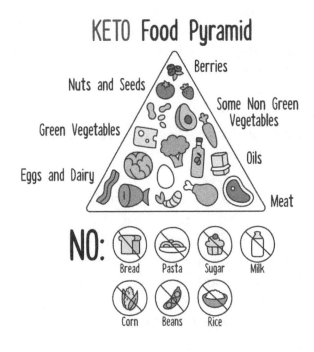

Looking at the standard ketosis diet, you find the ratio of 75 percent fat, 20 percent protein, and 5 percent carbohydrate. Since the diet has almost no carbs, it is essential to start with partial elimination in a week to help avoid those uncomfortable flu-like symptoms. Once you fully eliminate carbs, you can pursue the standard ketosis diet regularly to increase your autophagic performance and overall body health. Some of the foods you will need to avoid eating on the standard ketosis diet are:

- *Sugar*—sweets, candy, juice, soda, energy drinks, sugar additives

- *Grains*—bread, pasta, cereal, rice, etc.

- *Starchy Vegetables*—root vegetables like beets, carrots, parsnips, potatoes, yams

- *Legumes*—Lentils, beans, chickpeas, peas

- *Fruit*—all fruit except small amounts of berries

- *Unhealthy Fats*—canola oil, vegetable oil, margarine, Crisco

- *Some condiments*—condiments that contain any of the above ingredients and especially store-bought mayonnaise

- *Low-Fat food products*—any packaged food that is marketed as being low fat

- *Alcohol*

Foods that you can enjoy on the standard ketosis diet:

- *Meat*—grass-fed beef, pork, poultry

- *Fish*—salmon, cod, tilapia

- *Eggs*

- *Dairy*—butter, cream, some cheeses

- *Nuts* and *seeds*

- *Healthy oils*—olive oil, coconut oil, avocado oil

- *Avocados*

- *Low-Carb Vegetables*—leafy greens, lettuce, peppers, tomatoes, onion, cucumbers, asparagus

- *Herbs and Spices*—salt and pepper and a variety of herbs

The standard diet may seem like it contains very limited ingredients; however, these simple foods can be arranged in countless delicious ways, and there are several delicious recipes specifically for ketosis diets that support this style of eating to support you along the way.

The ratio of foods in the standard diet is that you would have the highest amount of fat, allowing your body to run on fat stores instead of carbohydrates. While burning fat and experiencing ketosis, you ensure a healthy amount of protein so that you don't start eating your muscular protein in the process.

The alternative to that is the high protein version in which you slightly decrease the amount of fat, and increase the amount of protein, leaving the carbohydrate intake the same. The fat ratio goes down to 60 percent with the protein up to 35 percent, leaving the last 5 out of 100 for the carbs. You may elect this method if losing muscle mass is of greater concern, or if you are working on building muscle through ketosis.

The important aspect of why ketosis diets work is that with the high fat-high protein approach, your body will always feel full and satisfied. You will not crave treats, carbs or sugars, especially if you start with partial-elimination of these foods before fully eliminating them from a standard ketosis diet. Many of the diets marketed today don't work because of this issue: cravings. Cravings break the diet and cause a return to the same patterns of insulin resistance and high blood sugar.

It is important that if you choose a ketosis diet for encouraging autophagy performance, you must not eat high fat-high carbohydrate-high sugar. This is the recipe for obesity, diabetes, and countless other diseases of the body.

The necessary program for you is something you will need to tweak along the way, depending on your level of physical activity and your overall goal for health. The ketosis diets are one part of a system that aids in the control of autophagy performance. As you start to incorporate this kind of diet, you can begin adding in intermittent fasts that will continue to offer your body greater opportunity to heal on a cellular level.

Ch 3.2: Steps to Water Fasting

Controlling autophagy can be easy and pleasant with the right approach. After reading about ketosis diets to get you on the right track for autophagy regarding food intake, you can now begin to introduce a greater autophagic response by starting a fast. Plan on giving yourself a couple of months on a new diet before diving into a fast. Allowing time for your body to adjust to anything is healthy. There are some serious key components to consider as well as some precautions and contraindications, before getting started with the steps to water fasting.

When you are considering your water fast, it is important to plan ahead. You don't want to wake up one morning and casually decide that today is the day you aren't going to eat and only drink water (unless you are sick and know that it is necessary). A healthy fast requires preparation and planning and the slow tapering off of food intake.

Figure 1: Intermittent fasting variants

Alternate-Day Fasting
(Eat over 12 hours; fast for 36 hours)

Sun	Mon	Tue	Wed	Thur	Fri	Sat
✗	✓	✗	✓	✗	✓	✗

Eat-Stop-Eat
(Fast or severely restrict calories for 24 hours, once or twice a week or just from time to time)

Sun	Mon	Tue	Wed	Thur	Fri	Sat
✓	✓	✗	✓	✗	✓	✓

Random Meal Skipping
(Randomly skip meals throughout the week)

	Sun	Mon	Tue	Wed	Thur	Fri	Sat
B -	✗	✓	✓	✓	✗	✓	✗
L -	✓	✗	✓	✓	✓	✓	✓
D -	✓	✓	✓	✗	✓	✓	✗

Feeding Window
(Eat only during a set period of time every day)

16- or 20-Hour Fast	8- or 4-Hour Eating Window

If you have never fasted, or water fasted before, start with only one day of water only, or try the 16:8 fast. If you are doing a 16:8 fast, you won't need to worry as much about the following steps.

Prepare by eliminating meals over the course of 2-3 days prior. Then, you can try one full day of water only. Giving yourself time to eliminate food slowly, before beginning a water fast helps to ensure that you won't suffer issues of fatigue, chronic headaches, nausea, and stomach cramping. Having enough water during a water fast, or any fast, is essential; however, too much water can disrupt your body's balance of sodium and potassium. A range of 10-14 glasses of water through the course of the day is recommended. As you gain comfort with one-day water fasting, you can then begin to allow for longer stretches once or twice a month.

From the one-day water fast, take it up to days and even three if you feel the need, or are prepared to handle that. If you start to feel symptoms of fasting like hunger or dizziness, drink a glass of water and rest. Be gentle with your body. Stand up slowly from sitting or lying positions and avoid strenuous activity and exercise. Meditation and yoga, or gentle stretching will be more appropriate during a water fast.

Attempting to exceed more than 3 days of water fasting may require consultation with a doctor or professional for guidance and aid. Consider what your goals and intentions are before excessive, long-term fasting. Mineral supplements and vitamins may be required for longer term fasts and can even be useful and helpful, in short term fasts. Some of the supplements you can consider using are not limited to the following:

- Sodium

- Potassium

- Magnesium

- Trace minerals

- Whey

- MTC oil (medium chain triglycerides)

- Nutritional yeast

- Collagen

There are some concerns and precautions for water fasting if you have certain medical conditions or diseases. Consult a doctor or professional before fasting if you have or suffer from any of the following:

- Advanced cancer

- Eating disorders

- High doses of prescription medication

- AIDS/HIV

- Alcoholism or drug addiction

- Advanced Type II Diabetes

- Advanced neurodegenerative disorders

If you are pregnant, or post-partum and breastfeeding, avoid water fasting and fasting in general for the health of you and your baby.

When you begin to plan your water fasting, there are some simple steps and guidelines to help you achieve the safest and healthiest autophagy performance. These steps are a good rule of thumb for any fast in general.

Steps and Guidelines for Water Fasting:

1. Plan water fasts when you will not be working and can have relaxing, restful periods.

2. Schedule it so you can first slowly eliminate food before transitioning to water only.

3. Schedule the length of the fast and plan what day you will slowly start to reintroduce food into your system.

4. Have the first foods available on hand before you start your water fast to prevent the need to drive to any grocery stores, in case you are feeling light-headed from the fast.

5. Choose clean, pure water, or distilled water only.

6. Fill containers of water to measure out how much you will need over the length of your fast. Try diving the measured water into to daily required amounts.

7. Reintroduce food with something simple and easy. If you are on a ketosis diet, make a smoothie of leafy greens, berries, and lemon juice, or eat a few spoonsful of high-fat yogurt. Keep it simple and small in quantity.

8. Gradually increase food intake slowly over a few days, avoiding processed foods or overly rich, decadent meals.

9. During the fast, be sure to enjoy lots of rest and relaxation. Do not overexert the body.

10. If feeling hungry, craving food, or having light-headedness, drink 1-2 glasses of water and rest for a while.

Controlling the process of healing on a deep cellular level requires some thought and planning. Engaging autophagy through water fasting can be healthy when approached in a healthy manner. Be sure to ease into a fast, slowly eliminating food, and ease out of it, slowly reintroducing food.

The benefits of water fasting are that you can clean, renew, refresh and restore your body while your internal intelligence cleans, renews, refreshes, and restores on the cellular level.

Ch 3.3: Weight Loss and Water Fasting

Hunger over the course of a water fast is greatly reduced when you start your fast off on the right foot. Energy may start off being lower during the fast, but the consumption of only water from 1-3 days restricts your caloric intake to allow for significant loss in weight. Because of the possible ketosis already occurring from the right diet, your body will already be burning fat stores over muscle allowing for healthy autophagic cell renewal.

What happens then is that during your short-term water fast, you are burning unwanted fat stores and flushing toxins from that stored fat with the water. The result is weight loss.

Loss of weight can get out of hand resulting in your body's instinct to control the loss of fat, hanging onto the reserves for survival. This can lead to taking energy from the protein stores in the body, which is why it is important to balance the fasting with the right diet, right exercise and right rest.

Fasting is believed to be one of the most effective ways to induce autophagy because of the entrance into a state of stress. The stress of this kind relates to the body's ability to engage all systems for survival. When these systems are over-engaged and out of hand, it can lead to severe illness; however, when done properly, recurring periods of timed stress can activate the body's ability to collect and remove waste for the optimal function that allows for survival. This is body intelligence.

Weight loss occurs when you fast, and water fasting actually enhances the ability to flush out what is needing to be released, adding to the overall loss of weight. Effects of fasting, when done properly lead to steady, regulated weight loss.

With the slow transition back to food, you are able to maintain the new weight and experience the rejuvenation on the cellular level caused by autophagy through fasting. There is no current evidence to suggest that weight loss is unhealthy through fasting. When one is properly prepared for a fast, there is less potential for harmful side effects. What you lose in weight, you gain in health.

Weight loss is one of the main reasons people fast. You don't have to water fast only to achieve significant weight loss. You can apply any of the methods of fasting revealed in Ch. 2.4 to promote weight loss; however, the results of water fasting, consuming only water for a period of time, creates a more profound impact on the initiation of autophagy and promotes the flushing of toxins and ketones from the body.

If the goal with water fasting is weight loss in addition to autophagy, be sure to allow time to phase into the right diet. Try incorporating a ketosis diet for 2-4 weeks, or more, before you begin to incorporate fasting. You may already begin to notice significant weight loss from the keto-diet alone. After a period of weeks, or months, you may hit a weight loss plateau and can use water fasting as a kick start to achieving more weight loss. Once you have regulated your diet in this way, you can begin to create a deeper autophagic response by slowly reducing food and calorie intake to enter into a fasting period. Again, you can determine the right fasting method for you by listening to your body, and paying careful attention to what works best for your body type, genetic history, and overall health.

Water fasting is an excellent method for promoting autophagic performance, which leads to healthy loss of weight that you can further maintain and regulate through right diet, exercise and rest.

Ch 3.4: Muscle Mass and Water Fasting

Marketing and advertising show that if you want to bulk up your muscles and keep hard-rock abs, you have to exercise all the time and pack in all the calories you can. Actually, you don't. It is no surprise that if you want to build muscle, you have to exercise, but unless you are a bodybuilder, or weight training for specific sports or athletic purposes, an exercise of various kinds a few times a week is enough to maintain healthy muscles.

Creating healthy eating habits is a must if you want a healthy body overall. If you eat hamburgers every day but go to the gym every day, you may believe that you are effectively utilizing the calories from that fast food meal to build muscle and feel healthy. Reports show that the kind of approach is like a dog chasing its tail. To truly benefit from both exercise and diet to build healthy muscles, a balance is required, as with all things in life.

Autophagy is part of a balance as well. Limiting your food intake for periods of time allows for the pendulum to swing so that your cells have the activity to repair themselves. If we do not create time and space for this, we are out of balance.

Many who consider autophagy as a long-term health plan for a long life and rejuvenation, may find concern about whether muscle mass is lost during fasting periods. This is a legitimate concern, and what water fasting contributes to is the activation of autophagy while resting the body.

During a fast, it is recommended to refrain from excessive exercise or overexertion. Those who have made a habit of exercising every day, may feel like they could lose muscle if they aren't working out at the gym on fasting days. While it would be supportive and healthy to do some light exercise and stretching, there isn't enough evidence to suggest that intermittent fasting can cause muscle loss, even when you aren't exercising. In fact, over exercise, while fasting is what could more likely lead to muscle loss.

The right health plan is entirely up to each person. Only you can know what is working or not working well by listening to your body. Periods of fasting regularly complimented by right diet, exercise, and rest can significantly improve overall muscle performance. When you are not fasting, you can be working on building your muscles through your regular exercise program. When you are fasting, you can modify your fitness routine to include less weight lifting and cardio, and more stretching, gentle resistance and deep breathing work. You can simply go for a walk around the neighborhood to engage your muscle groups while in a fasting period. Not all exercise needs to be powerlifting and cardio to support healthy muscular build.

With fasting, less is more, and balance is essential. There won't be a loss of muscle when water fasting; there will be activation of autophagic performance which leads to the prevention of many diseases, illnesses, and health disorders, and there will be a gain of optimal cellular function, rejuvenation of cells, and regulation of hormones and body systems.

Ch 3.5: Extended Water Fasting

Beyond the general promotion of autophagy through the right diet, exercise, fasting, and rest, there can be uses and reasons for extended fasting. Extended fasting may be something that lasts as little as 4-5 days or as much as weeks. Planning an extended fast means you probably have a good reason for it.

It could be regarded as a deeper healing measure for more chronic toxic release or disease reduction. It could also be intended for religious or political purposes that are based on personal beliefs, faith, and values. Other than that, for health, there are not a lot of reasons to explore extended water fasting. If you choose this method of autophagic performance, you will need to consult a medical professional or nutritionist who can provide some guidance and support.

There can be great dangers to the system as a whole with extended water fasting and seeking advice on mineral and vitamin supplements, and a scheduled plan for eliminating and reintroducing food is necessary for the healthiest benefit. Three to five days is doable when you want to cleanse, detox, and initiate autophagy. When you begin to exceed a week, you will need to have an appropriate support and plan in place.

The best method for prolonged or life-long autophagic performance is through intermittent fasting coupled with the right diet, exercise, and rest. Very sporadic, extended fasting may be useful for certain reasons, but consultation with a doctor or professional is advised for the healthiest experience.

Chapter 4: Optimizing Autophagy

The right diet, exercise, fasting, and rest are something you will know when you lock onto your need for autophagy. This need could alter over time, or it may be that you don't need every aspect of it in the same way for the rest of your life. All of the research on autophagy has shown that you don't need to do it every day, but you may find times in the course of your life that you will need or want to activate it on a daily basis. You may lose all the weight you set for your goal, using all four components, but will need to adjust your approach to autophagy once that goal is reached.

Life is long and changes daily. There will never be any diet, form of exercise, or fasting ritual that has to stay the same forever unless you are practicing these experiences for religious purposes. We grow, we transform, we change, for our whole lives and so should the food we eat, the kind of exercise we get, how often we fast, and what kind of rest is best under the circumstances.

We don't have the perfect relationship with these factors in a perfect way on all days of the year; we will ebb and flow and need to understand our responsibility to ourselves to pay attention, especially if you want to use autophagy regularly to enhance your health and renewal.

Significant research on the overall impact of prolonged autophagy has not been known yet; however, many improvements are being seen and experienced in the overall health of those who include performance autophagy activation in their regular health plans. You can guide yourself along the way using the ideas laid out in these chapters to help you determine the focus of your needs for inducing autophagy.

Bringing into focus all of the components of chapter 3, this chapter will outline the best methods for optimizing autophagy for deep cellular healing. Let your cells do the dirty work while you plan the routine, and handle the steps and instructions for initiating an autophagic response. Allow for some room to grow and shift. You don't have to follow these guidelines to a T; you can experiment and explore different ways of doing it that work best for your personal, optimal health.

Renewal is easy when you bring the right ingredients to the table. This chapter will give you the steps you need to change your diet, exercise, fasting routine, and resting time, in order to fully enhance autophagy. The four categories together promote the ideal healing platform. Remember, the recipe is in your hands, and you have the power to heal.

Ch 4.1: Right Diet

Taking what you know about how autophagy works and how to activate it, you can begin with the first important steps to creating that internal response. The next steps will give you the approach you need to shift and transition into the right diet. The right diet will initially be a keto-diet for the best autophagic response and weight loss, depending on your goals. A modified diet down the road will be beneficial as well; keeping your body healthy means listening and responding to its needs. A long-term keto diet can be adjusted to allow for more carbohydrates.

To begin a ketosis meal plan, you need to ease into it, like you would ease into a period of fasting. The reason for this is that when you immediately stop eating all the foods you are used to eating, such as bread, pasta, sugar, fruit, and many other items, you can enter a shock phase. For some, it can feel like illness, and there can be headaches, cravings, and fatigue. It can feel a lot like the flu. Your body has been eating certain foods for a while, and to suddenly deprive the body of these things can create an inflammatory response.

To create a smoother transition from your current eating habits to a keto-diet, you will need to break it down into phases and allow for some time. Week 1 will be the first phase of transition, eliminating some of the foods that you need to avoid to create ketosis. Week 2 will be the second phase of further elimination and increase in fat and protein. Here is a breakdown of what that may look like:

Phase 1: Elimination

- Alcohol

- Unhealthy fats like canola oil, vegetable oil, mayo, margarine, imitation butter

- All processed, low-fat foods

- Condiments containing sugars and carbs

- Most grains, including pasta, cereal, bread. You can keep small quantities of grains during phase 1, like rice, quinoa, and barley.

During this elimination, you are taking away some significant carbohydrates but are still allowed to eat some carbs and sugars found in fruit, starchy vegetables, legumes, and other sugary foods and beverages which will prevent a significant body shock. A possible weekly diet for Phase 1 could look like this:

Monday

> *Breakfast*: eggs and bacon with tomato and mushrooms

> *Lunch*: Salad with salmon and fruit on the side

> *Dinner*: Chicken soup with rice

Tuesday

> *Breakfast*: yogurt and berries with a tsp of honey and 3 tbsp of almond slivers

> *Lunch*: BLT on whole grain bread

> *Dinner*: Steak and potatoes with broccoli

Wednesday

> *Breakfast*: Fruit bowl with yogurt

> *Lunch*: Salad with chicken and quinoa

> *Dinner*: 3 bean soup with sausage and veggies

Thursday

> *Breakfast*: Goat cheese and basil omelet with tomatoes

> *Lunch*: Salmon and asparagus cooked in butter and lemon

> *Dinner*: Roast chicken with carrots and potatoes

Friday

> *Breakfast*: Poached eggs with tomatoes and kale

> *Lunch*: Codfish with steamed vegetables and butter

> *Dinner*: Beef Stew

Saturday

> *Breakfast*: Fruit and nuts

> *Lunch*: Turkey lettuce wraps

> *Dinner*: Roasted pork shoulder with vegetables

Sunday

> *Breakfast*: Eggs and bacon with a spinach feta salad

> *Lunch*: Salad niçoise

> *Dinner*: Baked Salmon and broccoli

This weekly diet starts to prepare you for an even bigger elimination of carbs and sugars, increasing fat and protein. Cooking with healthy fats like olive oil, coconut oil, and avocado oil is encouraged in Phase 1 and should be adhered to in Phase 2. You can also cook with a small amount of butter or clarified butter known as ghee.

There are many keto-diet cookbooks that contain specific cooking recipes to help you avoid incorporating any foods that you are working to eliminate. Avoidance of alcohol during phase one is important. Your body converts alcohol into sugar, so it is like drinking glasses or pints of candy. Increase water consumption and try more herbal teas. One of the reported side effects of ketosis is bad-breath. This is caused by ketones being released in the body from burning fat and can be evident in your breath. Rather than chewing sugary gum or sucking on sweet mints or lozenges, try a few cups of peppermint tea between meals. Adding freshly squeezed lemon juice to your glasses of water is a wonderful digestive aid and can help with balancing internal pH levels. You can also use apple cider vinegar in place of lemon juice to create the same effect.

Stay away from processed, packaged foods and try to prepare meals with fresh ingredients for the best results. Let go off all the protein and power bars, all the cookies and snacks, all the pastries and flavored lattes. Let go of all the bread and baked goods, all the food made with canola oil and corn syrup. This is what you begin to do in Phase 1. Give this phase some time. It doesn't have to be only one week. It may feel more comfortable for you to extend this phase into 2 weeks or more while your body adjusts. And be sure to drink plenty of water throughout.

Phase 2: Elimination

- All grains including any remaining bread, rice, quinoa, etc.

- All fruit, except small portions of berries

- All sugars and sugar additives, including honey and any beverage containing sugar

- Legumes—beans, chickpeas, etc.

- Starchy vegetables like beets, carrots, potatoes, yams and parsnips

During this elimination, you are further letting go of any remaining carbs and sugars. The standard ketosis diet allows for 5% daily intake of carbs in ratio to your fat and protein consumption. You can get these carbs from berries and some quantities of vegetables.

In Phase 2, you will be incorporating more of the high fat/high protein foods your body needs to stave off hunger and cravings, allowing your body to enter enhanced stages of weight loss and ketosis. A typical weekly diet with full elimination could look like this:

Monday

> *Breakfast*: spinach and goat cheese omelet with three eggs

> *Lunch*: tuna salad with feta, olive oil, and lots of leafy lettuce greens

> *Dinner*: pork chops with kale salad and broccoli

Tuesday

> *Breakfast*: yogurt and berries

> *Lunch*: big green salad with one avocado, cucumber, celery, green bell pepper, cabbage, toasted walnuts, and an olive oil lemon dressing

> *Dinner*: salmon and asparagus with butter and lemon

Wednesday

> *Breakfast*: bacon and eggs with tomato and basil, side salad

Lunch: guacamole with celery and cucumber sticks, a handful of nuts

Dinner: pesto chicken and roasted broccoli and brussels sprouts

Thursday

Breakfast: mushroom, spinach, tomato-basil omelet

Lunch: chicken salad lettuce wraps

Dinner: steak and eggs with salad

Friday

Breakfast: poached eggs on an arugula salad with feta and olive oil

Lunch: roasted pork loin and steamed veggies

Dinner: tilapia cooked in butter with sautéed broccoli, kale, and spinach

Saturday

Breakfast: yogurt and berries

Lunch: toasted nuts, one avocado, smoked salmon and celery sticks

Dinner: roasted turkey breast with a side salad

Sunday

Breakfast: omelet with scallions, mushrooms, cheddar

Lunch: salad niçoise

Dinner: roast chicken and brussels sprouts

Keep in mind that while cooking for a ketosis diet, if you need snacks between meals, eat nuts and seeds, or another kind of protein snack. Use healthy oils and clean ingredients. Do not use canned vegetables.

The Phase 2 diet has removed sugars, most carbs and increased proteins and healthy fats. Use ketosis recipes and cookbooks to help you adjust measurements based on your own weight and BMI. Additionally, if you are going to enjoy breakfast or snack items like yogurt and berries, be sure that you are choosing full-fat yogurt that does not contain any added sugars or flavorings.

Finding the right supplements for you can also improve the quality of your daily nutrient intake. Many herbal teas are packed with minerals, vitamins, and nutrients. Having a hot cup of tea between meals can stave off hunger, while soothing and warming the belly, helping it to feel full while packing in minerals and antioxidants.

Bone broth can be an excellent supplement to some meals as it is very filling and nutrient dense. Broths can also be useful in phasing out food to begin transitioning into a fasting period. Bone broths are simple and easy to make at home. You can purchase some quality bone broths from the store, but if you are cooking chicken for your ketosis diet, you can freeze the bones until you are ready to make broth and then put them in a crockpot overnight with purified water. Add some onion and celery for flavor. There are several recipes available for broths, and you can use a variety of bones, not just chicken.

Broths are soothing to the intestinal lining, providing a healthy space for nutrient absorption. Adding bone broths into your daily meals can be a huge improvement to your quality of digestion. You can have a cup of broth instead of tea or skip breakfast or dinner and just enjoy a cup of hot broth.

Finding ways to enjoy the program your body is undertaking can feel like a challenge at first, but initiating the process is part of the pleasure of starting your journey to healing. A cup of broth or a handful of your favorite nuts can go a long way.

Every person is different, weighs a different amount, and has a different health history. Finding the right recipes for you will help you feel like you can satisfy and satiate your hunger. Ketosis diets are in full, popular swing, and there are numerous delicious recipes to keep you on the right track. Engaging in a ketosis diet while enjoying some of the other autophagic activation methods will ensure a whole healing, whole body process.

Ch 4.2: Right Exercise

Get yourself ready to move your muscles. There isn't a time in your life when exercise will have no value or benefit. It is always a good idea to include exercise in your life. The limits of exercise depend on the person and the goals being worked toward; however, whatever exercise is chosen, you will add to the output of autophagy.

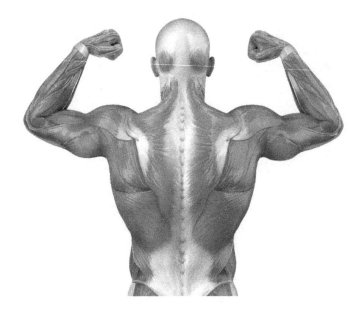

When you dial into the kind of exercise that works for your frame, build, performance goals, and intentions, you can expand on that exercise in various ways, creating the right routine for you. The key is finding something you enjoy. You don't have to program yourself to exercise like everyone else. In fact, that can cause burn out and avoidance. The right exercise is what is right for you.

Most exercise routines or plans promote some level of variety. This is essential to a balanced, physical health plan. What you choose depends on you, but within your routine, there should be a balance between resistance training or weights, cardio, balance, and stretching.

For optimal autophagy performance, there needs to be a flow within each of the methods. Doing the same exercise routine 6 days a week is not going to benefit anyone, long-term. Different muscle groups need time to recover and heal after the stress and strain of healthy exercise.

Here are some examples of some possible weekly workouts to promote autophagy:

Example 1:

Monday: Calisthenic Routine

Tuesday: Yoga

Wednesday: Weights

Thursday: Rest

Friday: Calisthenic Routine

Saturday: Yoga

Sunday: Walking with weights

Example 2:

Monday: Stretching for one hour

Tuesday: Barre/Pilates class

Wednesday: Rest and water fast

Thursday: Power walking with weights

Friday: Swimming Laps

Saturday: Rest and water fast

Sunday: Pilates

Example 3:

Monday: Weight lifting

Tuesday: Jogging for an hour

Wednesday: Rest and 18 hours fast

Thursday: Stretching and walking with weights

Friday: Swimming

Saturday: Rest and water fast

Sunday: Yoga

There are numerous ways you can plan an exercise routine, and if you begin to feel bored with it, you can change it! You may want to have a gym membership so that you have access to the equipment, machines and swimming pool, or you may prefer a home work out set up so you can easily exercise whenever you need to. You can acquire weight sets, stretch bands, yoga mats, and medicine balls to have available for use at any time. A little a day goes a long way.

Calisthenics

A majority of people today are aware of things like yoga, running, weight lifting, and all the different types of fat burning cardio workout you can find. Many people, though, are not as familiar with calisthenics. They are common enough exercises, but you may not have heard the name before. If you have heard of Cross Fit, then you understand calisthenics.

It is essentially a series of regular motor movements like standing squatting, walking, running, swinging, etc. that uses your own body weight for resistance and strength building. You really don't need a lot of machinery or equipment to use this kind of exercise. Many gyms offer training like this, providing a variety of different movements in a routine so that your whole body gets a full work out. You can also find several online videos that can guide you through a full calisthenic routine, many of which do not require any equipment.

Whatever method or schedule of exercise you choose, the right exercise is what is right for you, and all exercise will benefit your overall health, wellness, vitality and most importantly, autophagy.

Ch 4.3: Right Fasting

Not all the answers to health and wellness or weight loss and muscle health come from just diet and exercise. The connection that autophagy has to overall wellness and optimal body function, has been proven through research and studies over the past several years. A great number of autophagic performance results come from the practice of periodic fasting.

What can benefit you most during fasting is the planning and organizing of how and when you will fast for autophagic activation. There are several approaches to fasting and all of them can be useful at different times for different purposes. The ones that will be most effective for autophagy in combination with the right diet, exercise, and rest will allow for periods of time with no food at all and water consumption throughout. These periods can last as little as 16 hours or as long as three days. A common fasting practice is the 16:8 ratio. What this means is that you eat nothing for 16 hours and eat 2-3 meals within 8 hours. That could look something like this:

- 7 am—wake up and drink water and tea

- 12 pm—eat

- 3 pm—eat

- 7-8 pm eat

- 8 pm-12 pm the next day FAST

This is what daily fasting looks like, and depending on your hunger levels, you may only need two meals and a snack or just 1-2 meals. That is something you have to gauge on the day of the fast. This works well because your body is naturally in a fasting state when you sleep. When you wake up, instead of having breakfast right away, you wait until lunchtime to have your first meal and then have until 8 pm to satisfy your hunger. After 8 pm, you can drink water and herbal tea but will avoid food or snack, as well as alcohol. You can repeat this daily for continued benefit.

Another method of fasting that permits longer autophagic response is a longer fast, supported by healthy eating and transition on either side of the fast. An example of this type of fast can look like this:

Monday: skip breakfast, eat lunch and dinner

Tuesday: skip breakfast and lunch, eat dinner

Wednesday: very light dinner only

Thursday: water fast

Friday: water fast

Saturday: drink hot tea in the morning, broth midday, a small amount of yogurt

Sunday: broth in the morning, light lunch, light dinner

Monday: breakfast, lunch, and dinner

You can extend the length of the water fast to cover more days, or you can water fast for only one day out of the week, depending on your goals and intentions. You may find as you become familiar with the fasting experience that it is easy to shift back to food, without too much discomfort.

Another type of fast involves regular eating five days a week followed by 2 days of very light eating. You may not experience the most optimal autophagic response, but it will be activated by the extreme calorie reduction over the course of the 2 days.

When you decide how you want to fast, the right experience for you will be one that can occur at times where you can rest and not work, especially if you are water fasting. Incorporating the right diet and right exercise over the course of a week can look something like this:

Monday

> Breakfast: skip breakfast, *Pilates with weights*
>
> Lunch: tuna salad with feta, olive oil and lots of leafy lettuce greens
>
> Dinner: pork chops with kale salad and broccoli

Tuesday

> Breakfast: skip breakfast, *yoga*
>
> Lunch: skip lunch, water with lemon, and a cup of broth
>
> Dinner: salmon and asparagus with butter and lemon

Wednesday

> Breakfast: skip breakfast, water with lemon, *one-hour stretching*
>
> Lunch: skip lunch, herbal tea
>
> Dinner: salad (drink water throughout the day)

Thursday

> Water Fast: water throughout the day, *resting, meditation*

Friday

> Breakfast: skip breakfast, hot tea and *yin yoga*
>
> Lunch: hot broth, small salad with light dressing

Dinner: steamed vegetables with butter

Saturday

Breakfast: omelet with tomato and basil, *cardio workout*

Lunch: toasted nuts, one avocado, smoked salmon, and celery sticks

Dinner: roasted turkey breast with a side salad

Sunday

Breakfast: omelet with scallions, mushrooms, cheddar

Lunch: salad niçoise, *Calisthenics*

Dinner: roast chicken and brussels sprouts

You can repeat this fasting schedule every week and just play around with the recipes and exercise you do, or you can alternate weeks that you are fasting and do a 2-3 day fast twice a month.

The right fast for you is something to explore. Working to create optimal autophagy means allowing for periods of zero calorie intake, not just when you are asleep, so you can enjoy the maximum benefit of deep cellular healing. Find the fast that is right for your body. You may need to do some experimenting to make sure you can incorporate intermittent fasting into your lifestyle, diet, exercise, and rest.

Ch 4.4: Right Resting

Part of healing is allowing periods of time for your body to regenerate. Autophagy is a powerful, internal intelligence. Your body has the power to heal itself, but if you are not offering it the proper time to rest, you will be digging a deeper hole to clean up later.

Starting off on the right foot and creating good, healthy habits for wellness is essential to locking down the results you are looking for. In our current culture, everything is fast-paced, instantly gratified, and we are all plugged in all day long to our devices. Many people have 40-60 work weeks that make it challenging to find time for rest, let alone diet, exercise, and healthy fasting.

Bringing your health into focus includes allowing for proper periods of rest. During your experience in activating autophagy, it will be important to organize time for your body to rest. Rest is important after significant exercise. When you strain and stress your body, it requires time to recover and repair microscopic damage to the muscle fibers and tissues.

When you eat a meal that is filling, it is helpful to enjoy a period of rest after to allow your body the proper amount of time to digest. Your body can focus on digestion better if you offer it the rest to do so.

Fasting is something that can temporarily lower your energy since you are not ingesting any calories. It is common to experience some fatigue under these circumstances. It is a great opportunity to incorporate rest for your body while it is fasting. Imagine too, on the microscopic level, when you are resting your body is undergoing great healing, transformation and change, performing autophagic response from the intermittent fasting.

Many people consume large amounts of sugar and caffeine daily to bump them out of slumps that occur throughout the day, after meals, after long periods of work, or because of lack of sleep the night before. If you replace your caffeine and sugar doses with moments or periods of rest throughout the day, you would aid your body in a much healthier way, eliminating the need for caffeine and sugar altogether.

Sugar is the antithesis of a healthy diet and optimal autophagic performance and should be avoided anyway if you are planning on activating autophagy. Caffeine is regularly consumed by most people, and it is not discouraged in the majority of diets. The longer-term effects of daily caffeine intake can be as detrimental to your body as any other stimulant or toxin. Successful autophagic performance doesn't need caffeine and like other foods and beverages that hinder health. It should be avoided and replaced with herbal teas, water, and other non-caffeinated beverages.

You can ultimately rest better without it, and if you are getting the rest you need, you won't need caffeine at all.

The right rest comes with experimentation, awareness of your needs, listening to your body, and responding to it when it is asking for rest. Incorporating the right rest will fluctuate depending on day to day life, activities, exercise, diet, schedule, and more.

Rest is vital to supporting optimal autophagic performance. All four components together bring about a level of health, that will deliver clear results that you can see and feel. Activating autophagy through the combination of right diet, exercise, fasting, and rest is the key to a long and healthy life.

Chapter 5: Autophagy for Everyone

There is no one alive who doesn't have the internal intelligence to heal themselves. Creating a domino effect for autophagy to support a long and healthy life through the use of a certain diet, exercise and fasting is a choice you can make if you are ready. Activating this process is normal and is part of the inherent work of the basic human cell.

No matter where you are on your journey toward healing and healthy living, learning how to activate autophagy brings about a process of deep, cellular healing that renews and rejuvenates all the cells in your body preventing various diseases like diabetes, cardiovascular disease, neurodegenerative disease, and more. Other impacts involve the balance of hormones, healthier skin and hair, reduced inflammation, increased metabolism, stronger immunity, and revitalized cellular functions that allows for enhanced function in all body systems.

Transformation of the whole body occurs when you learn to activate the natural cleansing process all the way down to your cells. The focus of this book is to offer the reader information, understanding and steps to help begin this process on your own.

There are many studies and reports, testimonials and evidence to offer further details about the benefits of autophagy. This chapter will cover some of these topics, including frequently asked questions, myths, and endorsements from people's personal success with autophagy performance and health.

Ch 5.1: Frequently Asked Questions (Regarding Autophagy, Ketosis, and Fasting)

Question: What is autophagy?

Answer: Autophagy is a process on the cellular level by which cytoplasmic material such as dead organelles, oxidized proteins, and other scraps are transported to the lysosome in the cell for recycling.

Question: Why is autophagy beneficial?

Answer: It is a key process in a healthy functioning human body and is key to preventing diseases such as liver disease, various forms of cancer, neurodegenerative disease, autoimmune disease, and acute or chronic infection, to name a few. It also has a variety of anti-aging benefits because of the way it refreshes cells.

Question: Why do ketogenic diets promote autophagy?

Answer: Ketosis diets drastically reduce the intake of carbs to almost nothing and increase fat intake significantly which creates a drastic shift in energy, from glucose to ketones. This energy transition acts similarly to a fasting state, thereby leading to an increase in autophagic performance.

Question: How long does it take for autophagy to activate?

Answer: When glycogen is expended or drained through fasting, autophagy is activated, usually after 12-16 hours.

Question: If on a keto diet, how often should you intermittently fast?

Answer: Studies suggest that limiting long fasts to a few times a year can be beneficial, but that short 16-18-hour daily or weekly fasts are acceptable on a more regular basis and create more profound autophagy. It varies from person to person.

Question: Is fasting dangerous?

Answer: Fasting for 1-3 days is usually not a problem for healthy individuals. If you are not already on or working toward eating, a healthy diet, or if you have a chronic disease, such as liver, kidney, or heart disease, you may be at risk. Consulting a doctor before fasting is suggested if you are not sure if you are in a healthy state for it.

Question: How much weight loss can be expected with fasting?

Answer: It depends on many factors, such as how many calories you already eat a day, if you exercise and how long you are fasting. If you eat 2,000 calories a day, you may end up losing around 2-3 pounds on a 3-day fast. Losing more than that in a week could mean a loss of muscle rather than fat which is why healthy fasting is so important.

Question: How much will I lose with ketosis?

Answer: It depends on many factors, such as current weight and health, exercise, etc. On average, once your body starts ketosis, you may lose 1-6 pounds in the first week. After that, weight loss slows down to 1-2 pounds a week. If you are on a long-term ketosis diet, you will gradually lose weight more slowly. If you hit a plateau, it may be a good time to shake up your diet and branch out before returning to a standard ketosis diet.

Question: How do you increase autophagy?

Answer: Exercise. Fasting. Low carb diet.

Question: How often should I attempt intermittent fasts?

Answer: There are several methods, and you will have to find the one that feels right for you at the right time. Methods include 16 hours fasting/8 hours eating every day; % days regular diet/2 days fasting or restricted calorie intake; 24-hour fast 1-2 times a week; every other day fasting; fast all day and eat one big meal at night.

Ch 5.2: Myths About Autophagy

Myth: Fasting-induced autophagy causes starvation in the body.

Answer: Fasting is not starvation; it is taking a break from eating.

Myth: Autophagy eats away at your muscles when you fast.

Answer: Your body has ample resources in the form of glycogen and fat all over your body. If you are intermittently fasting, the first thing your body will do is go for the sugary glycogen, then the delicious fat before even considering the protein of muscle.

Myth: You will be malnourished if you fast to increase autophagy.

Answer: Fasting does not equal malnourishment, and as long as there aren't calories involved, minerals and vitamins are permitted if there is a concern of losing nutrients. Malnourishment is not attainable in a short-term fast unless you have a pre-existing medical condition.

Myth: The most important meal of the day is breakfast.

Answer: This slogan is propaganda from a time long gone. Scientific studies, advances in technology and research, and the experiences of many individuals have proven that is ok to skip breakfast.

Myth: Intermittent fasting is not good for your health.

Answer: Studies show that periodic fasting has numerous health benefits all of which relate to the activation of autophagy caused by fasting.

Myth: Keto diets are too high in fat and are bad for your heart.

Answer: Studies and research indicate that it isn't fat and cholesterol that cause heart problems; it is high carbohydrate, low-fat diets that create an unhealthy dynamic that leads to cardiovascular issues. Having high or low fat, high carb, and high sugar is the worse combination.

Myth: Keto diets allow you to eat all the butter, bacon, and steak that you want.

Answer: While ketosis diets are high in fat and protein, depending on your height, weight, and body mass index, it is important to regulate the amount of each based on your unique body profile. It won't be the same for everyone and unlimited bacon is not for everyone either.

Myth: Keto diets are the best way for anyone to lose weight.

Answer: No diet is perfect for everyone. Keto diets may not be right for you. All bodies are different, and so it is important to listen to your body to determine if keto diets are the best choice for you.

Myth: Fasting will cause hunger and overeating.

Answer: It isn't always a lack of food that causes hunger and overeating; it's eating too much all the time. Your body will always be expecting more sustenance on schedule, especially if you are always eating 3-square meals a day plus snacks in between. A lot of foods available are full of additives, preservatives, and sugar which you become addicted to and crave. Removing foods like this from the diet will dampen cravings and overeating. Fasting will create energy, vitality, and clarity.

Myth: Keto diets are a long-term solution.

Answer: While utilizing ketosis diets for weight loss and to promote autophagy can be beneficial, eventually you may need to find a more balanced solution. Your body will eventually need carbohydrates again for optimum health. Using keto diets periodically after a major weight loss, alternating with other healthy diet plans may be the best plan for long-term health.

Ch 5.3: Testimonials

"I have been overweight my whole life. Since I was a child, I ate food for comfort and was always heavy. I tried diets but ended up gaining weight in the process. A friend told me about her weight loss with ketosis diets and how it helps your cell regenerate in your body. The first few weeks, I lost 16 pounds with exercise and intermittent water fasting. I had never tried fasting or ketosis before and wasn't sure what to expect. It has been a year, and I have lost 38 pounds and feel wonderful. I still use water fasting periodically to help maintain my weight. I have so much energy, my skin is glowing, and I have more self-confidence about my health than I ever have in my life."

-Jeanine, 35

California

"I started bodybuilding in college going to the gym multiple times a week, eating a high carb, high protein diet to pack on the muscle. After a few years, I still wasn't at the level of weight training and muscle density that I wanted. Sometimes, I would feel a little sluggish before and after workouts. I saw a YouTube video about autophagy and how it can improve your health by cleaning the cells throughout the body. With the fitness programs and diet I was on, I learned that I needed to take it to the next level in my health outlook. I switched to a ketosis diet that allowed for some extra fat loss I needed which helped define my muscles. I started periodic water fasting and did carb intake on work out days only. The improvement in my muscles and energy was phenomenal, but I also felt great from the inside. No more sluggishness. It was like a light switch turned on, or my body got flushed and cleaned."

-Chad, 29

New York

"I tried a number of prescription drugs to help with my arthritis. They all seemed to work ok until I stopped taking them. I didn't like the side effects of taking them. I was never the sort of taking medication and have been healthy most of my life. I started looking for alternatives and discovered fasting with water only. I read several stories of people who were able to turn their inflammation around and live pain-free. I started with a trial fast to see how it felt, fasting and resting one day out of the week. I also cut out a lot of sugar, caffeine, and alcohol that were causing flare-ups in my arthritis. After a month of water fasting one day a week, I was able to stop taking the arthritis medication. I continue the fasts twice a month and have gotten rid of inflammatory foods and drinks from my diet. Now I can go on those long walks along the beach I enjoy so much."

Phillip, 63

Florida

"When I found out I had chronic fatigue syndrome, I was relieved to know what I had been struggling with in my health for the past few years. The downside was that none of the doctors seemed to have a cure for the symptoms. I started to do research online to see if any other people with chronic fatigue syndrome had had any success with medications or other methods. That's when I heard about autophagy. I began to change my diet and to exercise with a moderate routine three days a week. I started noticing a change right away when I tried a keto-diet, but it wasn't until I started fasting once a month that I really started to feel a big difference. It took several months of fine tuning my diet, exercise routine and when to fast, but now, a year and a half later, it is almost as if I cured myself of chronic fatigue."

Darcy, 42

Missouri

Conclusion

You are a living organism full of potential. You have everything you need within you to promote a healthy life. Changing your diet, exercise plan, and other factors is one thing; doing it to activate a deep, internal healing process is quite another. When you begin to look at the root cause of all the obesity, illness, stress, and short-lived lives, you can see that it is not just about what fitness and health magazines are promoting. You have to understand how your body is working hard to heal you from within.

In this book, you learned the basics of autophagy, what it is, and how it can literally change your health. You have also been given precautions, guidelines, and steps to activate autophagy in your own cells. It is happening on some level already, but you have the power to kick it into high gear to get the healing results you are looking for. You can renew, rejuvenate, and refresh your whole body with a few key components: right diet, right exercise, right fasting, and right rest.

Now that you have the knowledge of how to begin activating autophagy in your body, you can start making changes to help promote and support this process regularly. Try a few different ways and approaches and see what works best for your body. The right approach is just right for you. There is no diet or exercise program that is universally perfect, but autophagy is a part of us all. Start from there and watch your health transform.

Finally, if you found this book helpful or useful in any way, a review on Amazon is appreciated. Enjoy!

Image Bibliography

Human cell

http://www.slideplayer.com/slide/3858464

Lysosome

http://www.studyread/importance-of-lysosomes

Healthy vs Unhealthy Cells

http://dreamlifecrew.wordpress.com/2012/06/13/you-need-tre-en-en/unhealthy-cell

Autophagosome

http://nature.com/articles/ncb1007-1102

Types of Autophagy

http://novusbio.com/research-areas/autophagy

Ketosis

http://sites.bu.edu/ombs/2013/10/15/ketosis/

Insulin Resistance

http://adventistvegetariandiabetics.wordpress.com/diabetes-basics/articles-about-insulin-insulin-resistance

Keto Food Pyramid

http://universityhealthnews.com/daily/nutrition/keto-diet-health-benefits-of-ketogenic-diet/

Fast Schedule

http://examine.com/nutrition/the-low-down-on-intermittent-fasting/

Muscles

http://sciencedrivennutrition.com/caloric-restriction-and-your-muscles/